INTRAVITREAL INJECTIONS

A Handbook for Ophthalmic Nurse Practitioners
and Trainee Ophthalmologists

INTRAVITREAL INJECTIONS
A Handbook for Ophthalmic Nurse Practitioners and Trainee Ophthalmologists

Salman Waqar & Jonathan C. Park
South West Peninsula Deanery, UK

Michael D. Cole
Torbay General Hospital, Torbay, UK

Foreword by
Peter Simcock

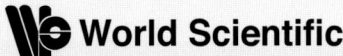

NEW JERSEY · LONDON · SINGAPORE · BEIJING · SHANGHAI · HONG KONG · TAIPEI · CHENNAI

Published by

World Scientific Publishing Co. Pte. Ltd.
5 Toh Tuck Link, Singapore 596224
USA office: 27 Warren Street, Suite 401-402, Hackensack, NJ 07601
UK office: 57 Shelton Street, Covent Garden, London WC2H 9HE

Library of Congress Cataloging-in-Publication Data
Waqar, Salman, 1970– author.
 Intravitreal injections : a handbook for ophthalmic nurse practitioners and trainee ophthalmologists / Salman Waqar and Jonathan C. Park, Michael D. Cole.
  p. ; cm.
 Includes bibliographical references and index.
 ISBN 978-9814571456 (pbk. : alk. paper) -- ISBN 9814571458 (pbk. : alk. paper)
 I. Park, Jonathan C., author. II. Cole, Michael D. (Michael David), author.
III. Title.
 [DNLM: 1. Eye Diseases--therapy--Handbooks. 2. Intravitreal Injections--methods--Handbooks. 3. Eye Diseases--nursing--Handbooks. 4. Intravitreal Injections--nursing--Handbooks. WW 39]
 RE959.5
 617.7'0232--dc23
                                                          2013043796

British Library Cataloguing-in-Publication Data
A catalogue record for this book is available from the British Library.

Copyright © 2014 by World Scientific Publishing Co. Pte. Ltd.

All rights reserved. This book, or parts thereof, may not be reproduced in any form or by any means, electronic or mechanical, including photocopying, recording or any information storage and retrieval system now known or to be invented, without written permission from the publisher.

For photocopying of material in this volume, please pay a copying fee through the Copyright Clearance Center, Inc., 222 Rosewood Drive, Danvers, MA 01923, USA. In this case permission to photocopy is not required from the publisher.

Typeset by Stallion Press
Email: enquiries@stallionpress.com

Printed in Singapore by Fuisland Offset Printing (S) Pte Ltd

CONTENTS

About the Authors	vii
Foreword	ix
Acknowledgements	xi
1 Introduction	1
2 Basics	3
3 Investigations	11
4 The Technique	29
5 Complications	41
6 Prototype Training Structure	53
7 Setting Up a Wetlab	59
8 Organising a Dedicated Clean Room	61
Further Reading	63
Appendix A: Intravitreal Injection Checklist	65
Appendix B: Basic Life Support Algorithm	68
Appendix C: Anaphylaxis Algorithm	69
Index	71

ABOUT THE AUTHORS

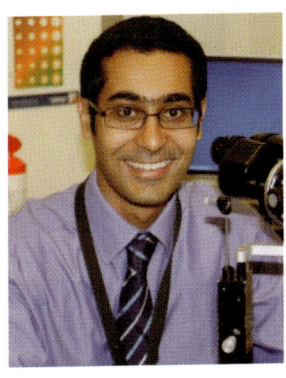

Salman Waqar completed his medical degree from the University of Health Sciences, Pakistan. He undertook basic training in general surgery (Sheffield) before joining an ophthalmology training programme in the beautiful south west of England. He has published extensively on the use of virtual reality training systems in ophthalmology and has also designed an interactive cataract surgery animation for patients (www.myeyesurgery.org.uk). He has regularly been involved with training ophthalmic nurse practitioners and is an instructor for the Basic Eye Surgical Training course held annually in Torbay. His prior foray into the world of books includes contributing to one related to ophthalmology training (refraction and retinoscopy).

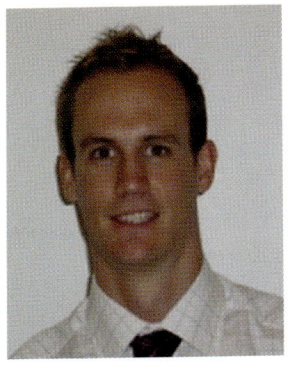

Jon Park graduated from the University of Bristol with degrees in Anatomical Sciences and Medicine & Surgery. Currently Jon works as an ophthalmic specialist registrar in the South West Peninsula Deanery and is the chief investigator for a nationwide study investigating sight threatening endophthalmitis following retinal surgery (in association with the Royal

College of Ophthalmologists' British Ophthalmic Surveillance Unit). He has previously authored a book related to training (refraction and retinoscopy) and several research papers related to the use of virtual reality surgical simulation as a training tool.

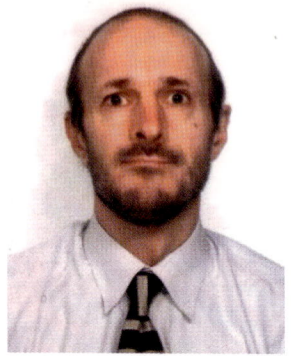

Mick Cole has recently retired as a consultant ophthalmologist after spending many dedicated years establishing a macular service at Torbay General Hospital.

FOREWORD

I am delighted to write a forward for this book which addresses the need to provide a detailed and clear account of how nurse practitioners should be trained to perform intravitreal injections in a controlled environment with patient safety paramount. This book provides a step-by-step approach starting with the basic anatomy and building to the technique itself whilst emphasising the awareness and management of complications. It also provides detailed guidance of how eye units should formally train nurse practitioners in this technique and ensure that all clinical governance issues that maintain patient safety are addressed. There is an ever increasing demand on eye unit resources to provide intravitreal injections not only to treat wet macular degeneration but also centre involved diabetic maculopathy and vein occlusions. A well-trained nurse practitioner can provide excellent technical expertise but also provides a continuity of care for these patients who usually require regular injections. The Royal College of Ophthalmologists and the Macular Society have recently supported the use of nurse practitioners for intravitreal injections and the authors are to be congratulated on a timely and well-written wealth of information for nurse practitioners which will also be useful for ophthalmologists in training.

Peter Simcock
Consultant Ophthalmologist
West of England Eye Unit, Exeter
June 2013

ACKNOWLEDGEMENTS

We are indebted to our lovely patient for her permission to photograph the procedure, to Sue Ashton (Ophthalmic Nurse Practitioner, Royal Eye Infirmary, Plymouth) who performed the injection, to Isabel Parry (Ophthalmic Nurse Practitioner, Musgrove Park Hospital, Taunton) for the idea to formalize our protocol as a handbook and to Khadijah Azhar for her beautiful illustrations. Our gratitude also to Mr Roger Gray and Mr Edward Herbert (Consultant Ophthalmologists, Musgrove Park Hospital, Taunton) for providing the excellent fundus fluorescein angiography (FFA) images.

1

INTRODUCTION

Age-related macular degeneration is the commonest cause of visual impairment registration in the UK. Intravitreal injections (injections into the vitreous gel of the eye) of anti-vascular endothelial growth factors (Anti-VEGF's) such as Lucentis® (ranibizumab), Avastin® (bevacizumab) and Eylea® (aflibercept) are now widely accepted to reduce the progression of "wet" macular degeneration. There is also good evidence of their efficacy in macular oedema secondary to diabetes and vein occlusions.

Ophthalmic nurse practitioners are increasingly becoming invaluable team members for delivering intravitreal injections particularly as the clinical demand increases. We have written this handbook to aid our nursing colleagues in such an endeavour and hope that it will provide concise but relevant information in a format that is easy to carry around and access. Towards the end we have outlined our experience with designing a training structure and it is our sincere hope that it will provide a framework for others too. We have extensive experience in organising wetlab sessions for both ophthalmic trainees and nurse practitioners and have added some easy tips for the readers to set up a session of their own. The appendices contain the latest information on Basic Life Support and anaphylaxis treatment. Whilst the nurse practitioner will always be in a well-supported environment and emergency response teams will be a phone call away, it is beneficial to be familiar with these algorithms. The book is aimed primarily at nurse practitioners but we are confident that it will also be a useful reference for junior ophthalmic trainees learning how to perform intravitreal injections.

We wish you all the best for your career as part of the retinal team!

Salman Waqar
Jon Park
Mick Cole

2

BASICS

In order to be proficient in intravitreal injections, it is crucial to appreciate the structure of the eye and how this knowledge can be used to give a safe injection.

The eye is a highly specialised organ of photoreception, a process by which light energy from the environment produces changes in specialised nerve cells in the retina (rods and cones). These changes result in action potentials (the electrical voltage across a cell) which are subsequently relayed to the optic nerve and then to the brain where the information is processed and consciously appreciated as vision.

The eye is an approximate sphere 2.5 cm in diameter (equivalent to an axial length of 25 mm), with a volume of 5 mL (fills 1/6th of the orbit whose volume is 30 mL). The eye consists of 3 basic layers.

THE THREE LAYERS OF THE EYE

1. **The fibrous corneoscleral coat** consisting of the cornea and sclera.

- **The Cornea**

This is the anterior most transparent window of the eye. The cornea meets the sclera at the limbus, which is also where the

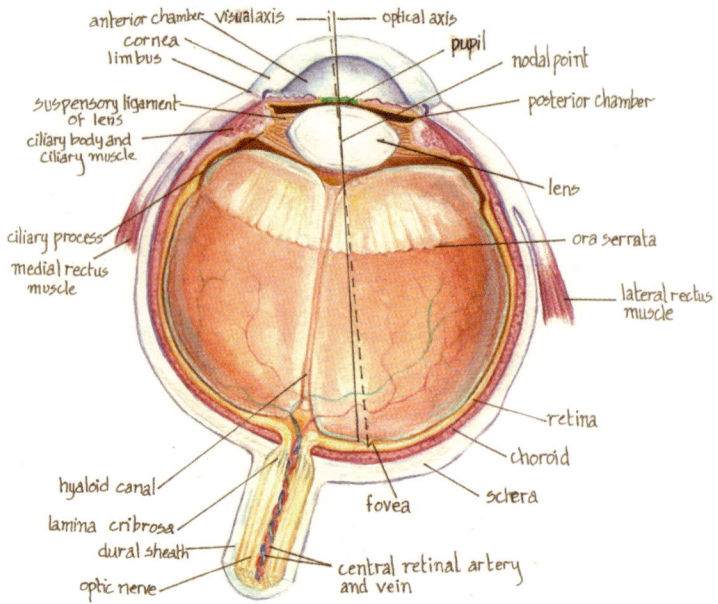

Fig. 2.1. The eye in cross section.

conjunctiva ends. The conjunctiva covers the sclera but does not cover the cornea. The cornea is kept transparent by its avascularity and the innermost monolayer of cells (endothelium) which pumps fluid out of the corneal stroma. The cornea presents a tough barrier to trauma and infection and is responsible for about 2/3rd of the eyes' refractive power (the other 1/3rd coming from the lens).

- **The Sclera**

This is an opaque white fibrous coat which also protects the eye and maintains its shape due to inherent structural integrity.

2. **The uvea (or uveal tract)** which is the middle vascular pigmented layer of the eye and consists of the iris, ciliary body and choroid.

- **The Iris**

This is a thin contractile circular disc which is analogous to the diaphragm of a camera. The iris separates the anterior and posterior chambers which are filled with aqueous humour and are in continuity through an opening, the pupil. The iris is attached by its root at the "angle" (iridocorneal) of the anterior chamber where it merges with the ciliary body and trabecular meshwork. Aqueous humour drains mainly through the trabecular meshwork which is visible using a mirror within a contact lens called a gonioscope.

- **The Ciliary Body**

This is approximately 6 mm in width and is responsible for the production of aqueous humour. It also contains muscles which are attached to the zonular ligaments of the lens (changing its shape on contraction to focus or accommodate). It has two parts, the pars plicata and the pars plana. The pars plicata is the anterior part. It is 2 mm long (measured from the limbus) and contains about 70 ciliary processes which are the site of attachment for the aforementioned zonular ligaments. The pars plana is a posterior flat area 4 mm long. As the sclera and cornea are relatively rigid, excess production/reduced drainage of aqueous humour or injection of substances into the eye leads to raised intraocular pressure (normal is up to 21 mmHg). Intraocular pressure is high immediately after intravitreal injections (can be as high as 60 mmHg). Normalisation of the pressure usually occurs over 30 min after injection and is dependent on aqueous humour outflow through the trabecular meshwork. The safest site for administering intravitreal injections is through the pars plana. This is because it lies behind the lens and in front of the retina, thus avoiding damage to either of these structures.

- **The Choroid**

This highly pigmented and vascular posterior portion lies between the sclera and the retina and extends forward to the ciliary body. Its principal function is to nourish the outer layers of the retina and prevent unwanted light from reflecting back through the retina. It is composed of an outer layer of large calibre blood vessels which divide into smaller diameter vessels and ultimately form the choriocapillaris (a network of capillaries). These drain into the vortex veins which ultimately drain into the superior and inferior ophthalmic veins. The innermost layer of the choroid is a membrane called the Bruch's membrane. The basal portion of the retinal pigment epithelium (RPE) is attached to this membrane. This is of clinical importance as in age-related macular degeneration (AMD) it is the Bruch's membrane that is breached by abnormal choroidal blood vessels, leading to pathognomic features of the disease (as discussed later in the imaging section).

3. The retina (neural layer) this is where photoreception occurs and consists of two primary layers, the inner neurosensory retina and an outer layer called the retinal pigment epithelium. Anatomically the following regions are described:

- **The macula** (Latin "patch") (same as macula lutea) is the area within the main vascular arcades and is 5–6 mm in diameter. Cone photoreceptors are mostly concentrated here for fine resolution (maximum density in the fovea).
- **The fovea** (Latin "pit") is the central 1.5 mm diameter area of the macula. The foveola is the central 0.35 mm diameter area of the fovea (Fig. 2.2)
- **The optic disc** is 1.5 mm in diameter. It contains no normal retinal layers or photoreceptors (thus causing the blind spot) and is the area where nerve fibres of the retinal ganglion cells pierce the sclera to enter the optic nerve. The central pale thinned area of the disc forms the cup, which becomes progressively enlarged through loss of ganglion cells in glaucoma. The cup's vertical diameter is measured in relation to the disc diameter when monitoring patients with glaucoma (referred to as the cup to disc ratio).
- **The peripheral retina** is rich in rod photoreceptors which provide acuity in low levels of illumination.

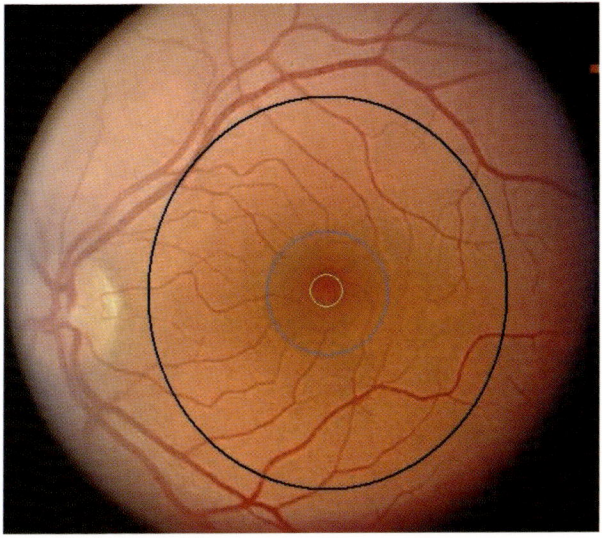

Fig. 2.2. A normal fundus photograph (left eye) showing the approximate locations of the macula (black circle), fovea (blue circle) and foveola (green circle).

- **The ora serrata** is where the peripheral retina ends. This is approximately 7 mm from the limbus.

The Retina in Cross Section

The retina consists of 10 layers. From posterior to anterior these are (Fig. 2.3):

1. **Retinal pigment epithelium (RPE).** A monolayer of cells which have several functions, including maintaining the adhesion of the neurosensory retina, rendering the sub-retinal space dry, removing shed portions of photoreceptor outer segments, contributing to the transport and storage of metabolites/vitamins and providing a blood retinal permeability barrier.
2. **Photoreceptor layer.** This contains rod and cone inner/outer segments. The outer segments contain the visual pigments that are responsible for absorption of light and initiation of the neuroelectrical impulse, whilst the inner

8 ♦ *Intravitreal Injections*

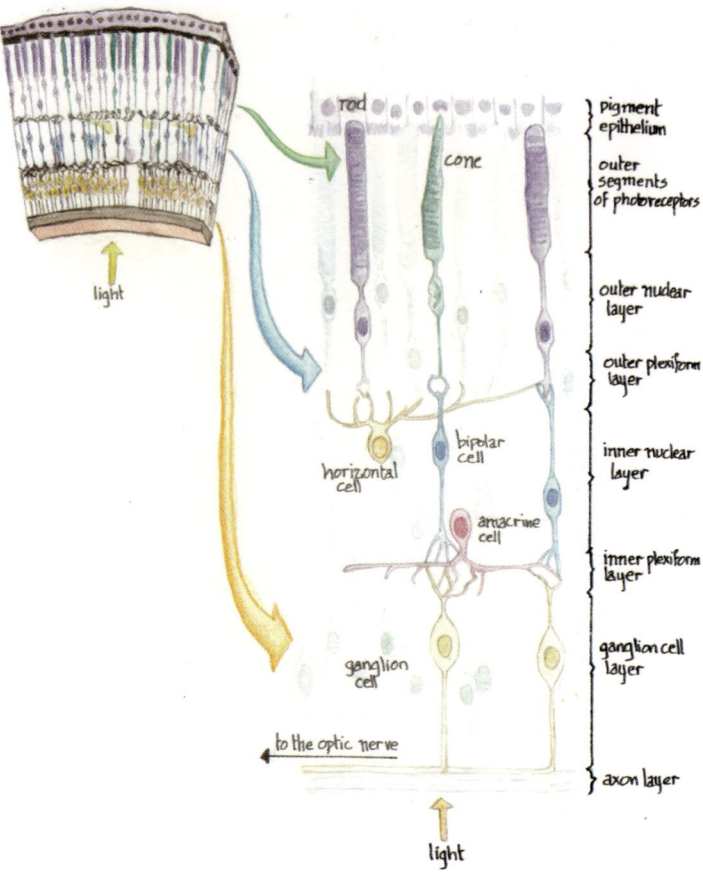

Fig. 2.3. The retina in cross section.

segments contain the cellular apparatus required to provide energy, e.g. mitochondria. The junction of the two segments is visible on high resolution OCT as discussed later.
3. **External limiting membrane.** The external limiting membrane is a histological feature of the retina and is a dark line caused by junctions between photoreceptors and muller cells. It is located between the photoreceptor and outer nuclear layers.
4. **Outer Nuclear Layer.** This contains the nucleated cell bodies of the rods and cones. Cones subserve fine resolution

essential for reading, spatial resolution and colour vision whilst rods sense contrast, brightness and motion. Rods are also mainly responsible for peripheral and night vision.
5. **Outer Plexiform Layer.** This contains the cone and rod axons as well as dendrites of horizontal bipolar cells.
6. **Inner Nuclear Layer.** This contains the nuclei of horizontal cells, bipolar cells, amacrine cells and muller cells.
7. **Inner Plexiform Layer.** This contains the axons of bipolar cells and amacrine cells along with dendrites of ganglion cells.
8. **Ganglion Cell Layer.** This contains the nuclei of the ganglion cells.
9. **Nerve Fibre Layer (Axon Layer).** This is formed by the axons of ganglion cells traversing the retina to leave the eye at the optic disc.
10. **Inner Limiting Membrane.** This is a membrane on the inner surface of the retina.

The Vitreous

The vitreous is a thick, transparent substance that fills the centre of the eye between the lens and the retina. It is composed mainly of water and constitutes about 2/3rd of the eye's volume. The viscous properties of the vitreous allow the eye to return to its normal shape if compressed.

In children, the vitreous has a consistency similar to an egg white. With age it gradually thins and becomes more liquid. The vitreous is firmly attached to certain areas of the retina. As the vitreous thins, it separates from the retina, often causing floaters. This may ultimately lead to separation from areas around the optic disc and retinal periphery (a condition called posterior vitreous detachment or PVD). There are various causes of retinal detachment (detachment of the neurosensory retina from the RPE), but the commonest cause is due to pulling forces on the peripheral retina by the posterior lining of the vitreous at the time of a PVD. Fortunately, most PVDs do not result in retinal detachments, since although PVD is common, retinal detachment is relatively rare. PVD itself is not sight threatening but if associated with a retinal detachment, treatment is typically required to prevent loss of sight. During intravitreal injections, incorrect placement of the needle through the retina can cause a tear and lead to a retinal detachment too.

The Lens

In addition to appreciating the three layers of the eye, knowledge of the lens is also important to avoid inadvertent damage.

The lens is a highly organised system of specialised cells within a transparent capsule. Situated in the anterior segment of the eye, it provides a third of the refractive power of the eye. Zonules from the ciliary body hold the lens in place.

A cataract (Latin for "waterfall") is regarded as a visually significant opaqueness of the lens for which age is the most common risk factor. Cataract surgery is the commonest operation performed in the UK. Damage by a needle during an intravitreal injection can lead to rapid cataract development and problems due to sudden swelling of the lens.

3

INVESTIGATIONS

Every patient presenting for an intravitreal injection will have gone through an investigative process in clinic. The ophthalmic nurse practitioner will inevitably come across the results of these either in clinic or whilst looking through the notes prior to injecting. Also nurse practitioners are now increasingly reviewing patients in clinics and may in the future be an integral part of "virtual" clinics where they will carry out investigations at a peripheral site and the clinician will review the results in hospital. Therefore, an understanding of the basic investigative techniques employed is beneficial. Here we discuss the essentials of Optical Coherence Tomography and Fundus Fluorescein Angiography.

OPTICAL COHERENCE TOMOGRAPHY (OCT)

OCT allows high-resolution cross-sectional (tomographic) images of the retina to be obtained in a non-invasive manner. It works by measuring the properties of light waves reflected from tissue (similar to sound wave measurements in ultrasonography). However, the utilization of light instead of sound presents a technical challenge. The speed of light makes direct measurements on the reflected waves impossible. In OCT systems, this hurdle is overcome through the use of a technique called interferometry. In interferometry, a beam of light is divided into a measuring beam and a reference beam. The reconvergence of light reflected from the tissue of interest and light reflected from a reference path produces characteristic patterns of interference that are dependent on the mismatch between the reflected waves (Fig. 3.1). Because the time delay and amplitude of one of the waves (i.e. the reference path) is known, the time delay and intensity of light returning from the sample tissue may then be extracted from the interference pattern. A two-dimensional or three-dimensional image of the retina is then created in which "hot" colours denote stronger reflectivity and "cool" colours denote weaker reflectively. Thus, highly reflective tissue is reddish-white, whereas less reflective tissue is bluish-black. Alternatively, the OCT image can be displayed on a gray scale where more highly reflected light is brighter than less highly reflected light.

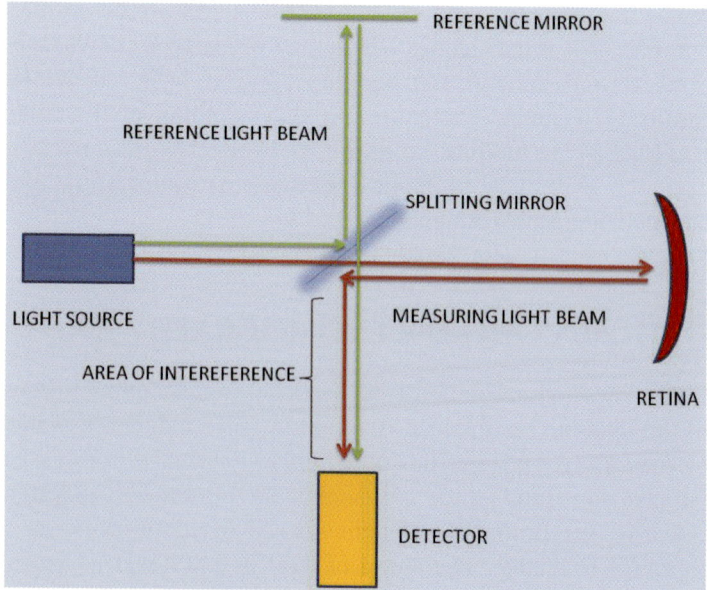

Fig. 3.1. Schematic diagram of a Michelson interferometer demonstrating the principle of optical coherence tomography.

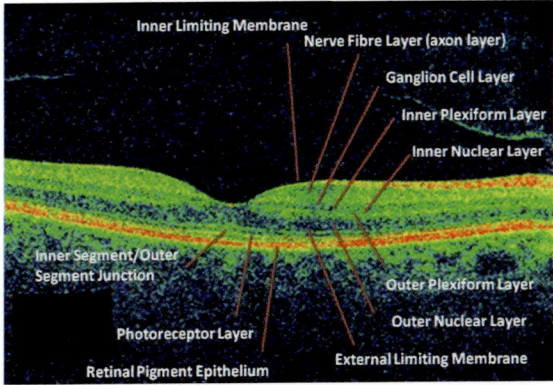

Fig. 3.2. A normal spectral domain OCT showing an approximate correlation of the anatomical layers. Notice the higher resolution as compared to time domain systems.

The first hyper-reflective layer detected is the internal limiting membrane (ILM). The retinal nerve fibre layer and both the inner and outer plexiform layers are seen as hyper-reflective. The ganglion cell layer and both the inner and outer nuclear layers are hypo-reflective. Within the photoreceptor layer, the external limiting membrane and the junction of the inner/outer segments are hyper-reflective. The RPE appears hyper-reflective too (Fig. 3.2).

There are two types of OCT scan machines:

1. Time domain OCT. This is the older generation of OCT scan machines. Here, interference patterns are assessed as a function of time and therefore the resolution is low and it takes longer to acquire an image (able to visualise structures down to 10 µm and acquire images at a rate of 400 scans per sec) (Fig. 3.3).
2. Spectral domain OCT. These newer generation systems use spectral interferometry and a mathematical function called Fourier transformation to assess interference patterns as a function of frequency rather than time. This allows light scattered from different depths within the tissue to be measured simultaneously.

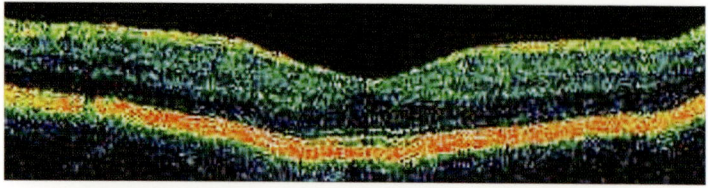

Fig. 3.3. A time domain OCT of a normal macula.

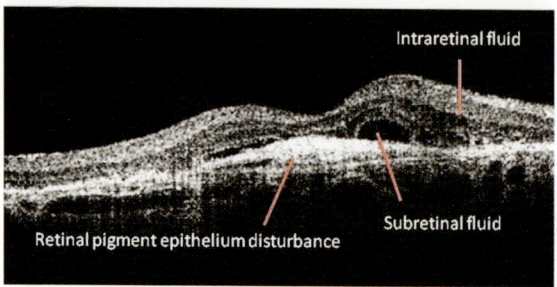

Fig. 3.4. Spectral domain OCT scan of an eye with wet age related macular degeneration (choroidal neovascularisation) showing intraretinal fluid, subretinal fluid and RPE disturbance.

In simple terms, images can be acquired more quickly than in time domain systems (over 20,000 scans per sec) and the resolution is higher (able to visualise structures down to 3 μm).

Common pathological appearances seen on an OCT scan are:

1. Choroidal neovascularisation (CNV) or "wet" age-related macular degeneration (AMD) is caused by abnormal choroidal blood vessels breaking through the RPE. An OCT scan will show a RPE disturbance, subretinal and intraretinal fluid as shown (Fig. 3.4).
2. A pigment epithelial detachment (PED) can be seen in both "dry" and "wet" AMD. In the dry instance, deposition of abnormal degenerative material (drusen) between the RPE and the Bruch's membrane causes the RPE to detach, resulting in a dome-shaped elevation as shown (Fig. 3.5).This is called a serous PED. A PED can also be seen in a form of wet

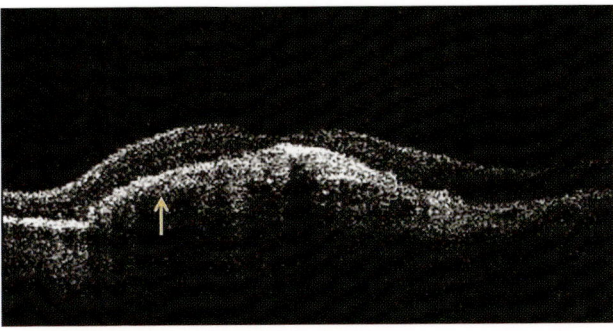

Fig. 3.5. OCT showing a PED (arrow). Note the dome shaped elevation of the retinal pigment epithelium.

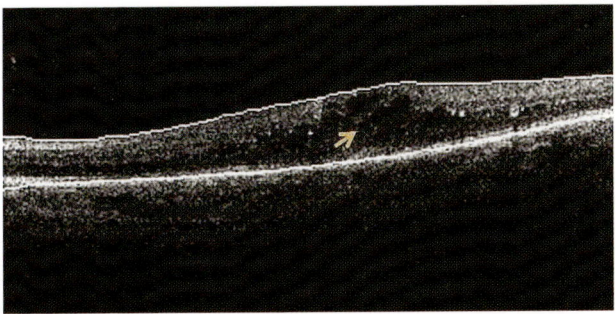

Fig. 3.6. OCT scan showing cystic intraretinal spaces consistent with cystoid macular oedema (arrow).

AMD (called occult CNV), where abnormal choroidal blood vessels are present between the Bruch's membrane and the RPE, again causing the RPE to detach. This is called a fibrovascular PED. It is not possible to differentiate between the two kinds of PEDs based on OCT alone. A combination of fundoscopy, OCT and fluorescein angiography can help reach a diagnosis.
3. Cystoid macular oedema can be seen in eyes with inflammation (uveitis) or following a vein occlusion. This presents as cystic spaces within the retina as shown (Fig. 3.6).
4. Diabetic macular oedema presents simply as intraretinal fluid (Fig. 3.7).

16 ♦ *Intravitreal Injections*

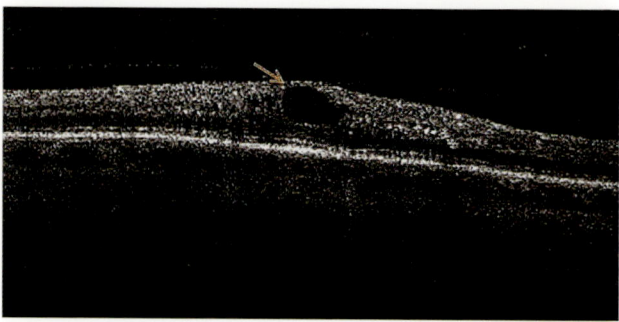

Fig. 3.7. OCT scan in a diabetic patient showing intraretinal fluid (arrow) indicative of diabetic macular oedema.

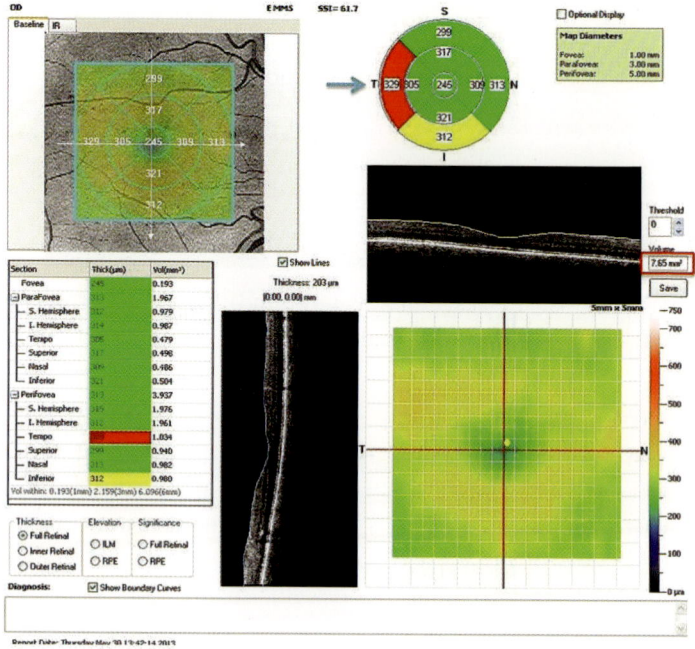

Fig. 3.8. A full page report of a normal OCT (right eye). Such reports provide various other useful parameters for serial monitoring in addition to a retinal cross section. Macular volume (red box) and numerical values of macular thickness (blue arrow) are particularly useful.

> **Further reading**
>
> Further information on the science of OCT scans can be gained from these articles which we have referenced from:
>
> 1. Jaffe GJ, Caprioli J. (2004) Optical coherence tomography to detect and manage retinal disease and glaucoma. *Am J Ophthalmol* **137**(1):156–69.
> 2. Keane PA, Patel PJ, Liakopoulos S, *et al.* (2012). Evaluation of age-related macular degeneration with optical coherence tomography. *Surv Ophthalmol* **57**(5): 389–414.

FUNDUS FLUORESCEIN ANGIOGRAPHY (FFA)

This technique involves intravenously injecting a dye (fluorescein sodium) to allow visualisation of the retinal and choroidal circulation alongside any associated abnormalities. Fluorescence is the property of certain substances to emit a light of longer wavelength when stimulated by light of a lower wavelength. Fluorescein sodium is excited by blue light (490 nm) and emits yellow-green light (530 nm). It is water-soluble and once within the circulation, approximately 80% of it is bound to plasma proteins whilst the rest remains unbound. Its passage through the retinal and choroidal circulation follows certain anatomical principles which are:

- The choriocapillaris (the smallest blood vessels in the choroid) are permeable to the unbound fluorescein. This leaks out and passes through the Bruch's membrane but cannot pass through the retinal pigment epithelium. Tight junctions here prevent any further passage and this forms the "outer blood–retinal barrier."
- The retinal blood vessels have tight junctions, too, that prevent any fluorescein (both bound and unbound) to pass out. This is called the "inner blood–retinal barrier."

Usually 5 mL of 10% fluorescein sodium is injected as a bolus intravenously. A cobalt blue excitation filter attached to

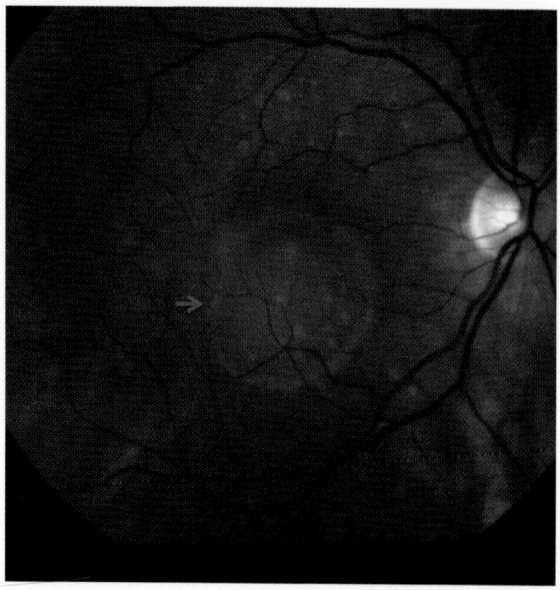

Fig. 3.9. Red free image. A localised retinal disturbance can be seen (arrow).

the camera allows only blue light to reach the retina. The fluorescein is excited and only yellow-green light is allowed back to the camera via a yellow green barrier filter. A wide gauge cannula should ideally be inserted, as this will be invaluable for management should treatment be needed for anaphylaxis. A red free image is usually taken prior to injecting fluorescein. This is done with a yellow-green filter in place, thus blocking red light. As a result, red structures appear black allowing better visualisation of any vascular abnormalities. Localised retinal structural abnormalities can also become more evident (Fig. 3.9).

A normal FFA demonstrates the following well recognised phases:

1. Pre-arterial or choroidal phase. It takes approximately 10 to 15 sec for the fluorescein to reach the eye following

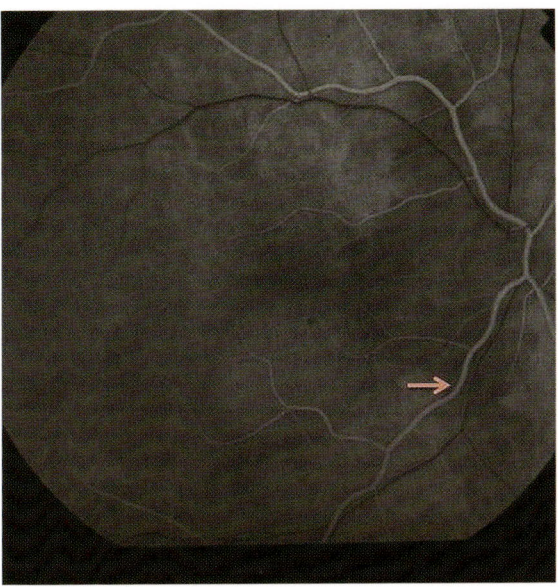

Fig. 3.10. FFA showing arterial filling with fluorescein sodium dye (arrow).

injection. This can be longer in patients with systemic disorders causing circulatory insufficiency, e.g. atherosclerosis. Once in the eye, it enters the choroidal circulation a second earlier than the retinal circulation. Thus, the first phase presents a diffuse leakage of dye from the choriocapillaris known as a "choroidal flush." The choroid appears fluorescent but there is no dye yet in the retinal vessels.

2. Arterial phase. As the name implies this phase shows the retinal arteries filling up with dye a second or so after the choroidal phase (Fig. 3.10).
3. Arteriovenous phase. In this phase the veins begin to show laminar flow (Fig. 3.11). This means that the dye is flowing adjacent to the venous walls initially due to faster plasma flow adjacent to the vessel wall.
4. Venous phase. During this phase the veins fill up completely with fluorescein (Fig. 3.12). The fovea remains dark due to:

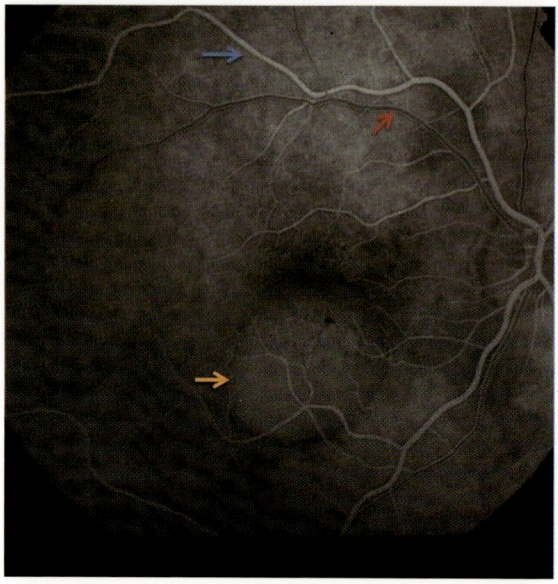

Fig. 3.11. FFA showing arteries filled up (blue arrow) with laminar venous flow (red arrow). Note the localised dye pooling (orange arrow) indicating a pigment epithelial detachment. This is a pathological finding and would not be expected in a normal FFA.

- absent blood vessels (this is also called the foveal avascular zone).
- high density of the pigment xanthophyll blocking the background choroidal fluorescence.
- larger RPE cells with higher concentrations of pigments melanin and lipofuscin blocking the background choroidal fluorescence.

By now around 30 sec have passed since dye injection and its first pass through the eye is complete.

5. Late phase. This is also called the recirculation phase. Here the dye continuously recirculates through the eye, the fluorescence getting less intense as time passes until it is completely

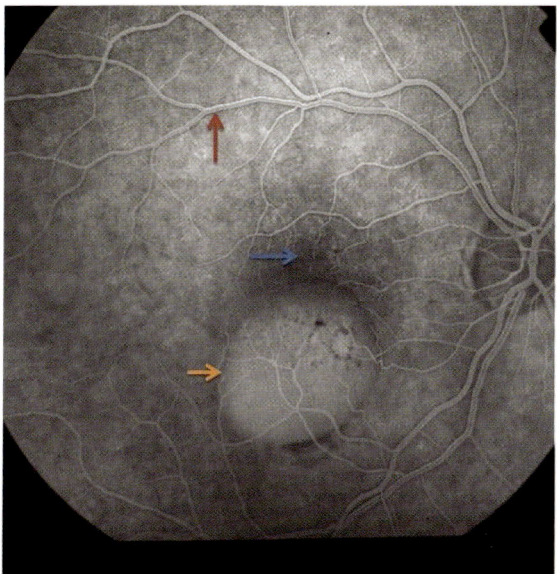

Fig. 3.12. Venous phase showing complete venous filling (red arrow). The fovea is dark (blue arrow). A localised subretinal pooling of dye (orange arrow) indicates a pigment epithelial detachment. This is a pathological finding and would not be expected in a normal FFA.

absent by around 10 min. The optic disc continues to show staining for a while afterwards. Sometimes the preceding four phases are collectively referred to as the early phase.

FFAs are interpreted in terms of areas of increased and decreased fluorescence. These are called hyperfluorescent and hypofluorescent, respectively. Whilst looking at a FFA image, one can tell which eye the image is from by ascertaining which side the optic disc is on, i.e. if the optic disc is on the right side of the image then we are looking at a FFA of the right eye and vice versa. Areas of hyperfluorescence are seen in the following conditions:

- Leakage of the dye as is seen in choroidal neovascularisation (Figs. 3.13, 3.14 and 3.15).This is one of the most common

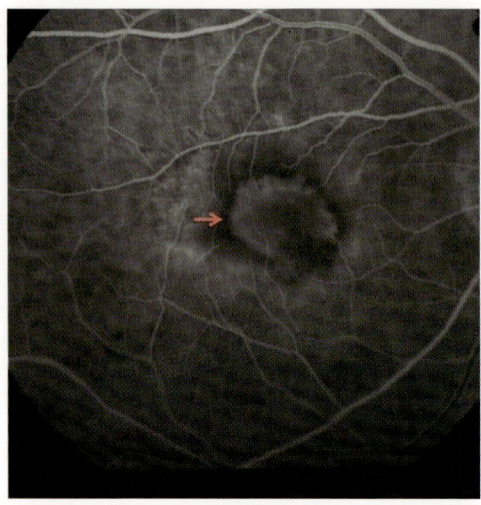

Fig. 3.13. FFA showing early hyperfluorescence (within 30 sec) indicative of "classic" choroidal neovascularisation. The appearance is often described as having a "lacy" pattern.

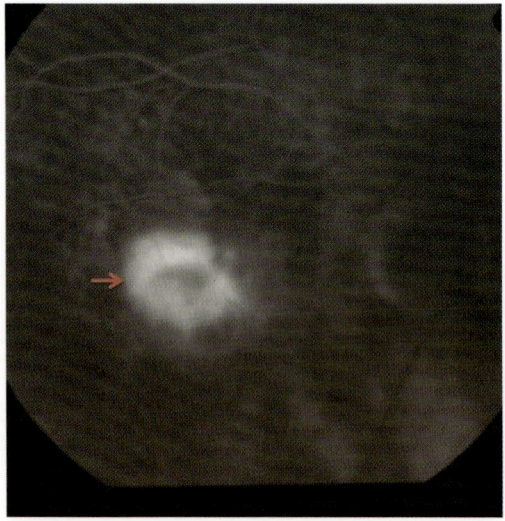

Fig. 3.14. FFA of same eye showing increase in intensity and area of the hyperfluorescent area in the late phase (at 3 min). This confirms the presence of "classic" choroidal neovascularisation.

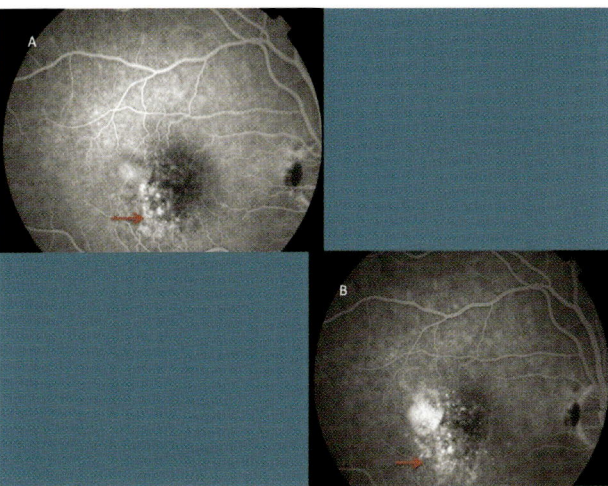

Fig. 3.15. FFA showing late hyperfluorescence at approximately 40 sec as indicated by red arrow (image A). The area increases in intensity and size in the late phase at approximately 3 min (image B). The appearance is "stippled" and this is characteristic of "occult" choroidal neovascularisation.

indications for anti-VEGF intravitreal injections. Leakage can also be seen in cystoid macular oedema which can occur following a branch or central retinal vein occlusion (Fig. 3.16). Similarly, diabetic macular oedema is characterised by diffuse hyperfluorescence (Fig. 3.17). Intravitreal anti-VEGF or steroid injections may be used to treat these conditions as well.

- "Window defects" refer to areas where choroidal fluorescence becomes more visible due to a defect in the RPE. This can be seen in areas of RPE atrophy secondary to dry age-related macular degeneration (Figs. 3.18 and 3.19).
- Pooling refers to accumulation of fluorescein dye into an anatomical space that may have increased in size due to a pathological process. A common example is a retinal pigment epithelial detachment (PED), the mechanism of which has been discussed in the OCT section. On a FFA, this presents as an early well-defined filling of fluorescein under the detached

24 ♦ *Intravitreal Injections*

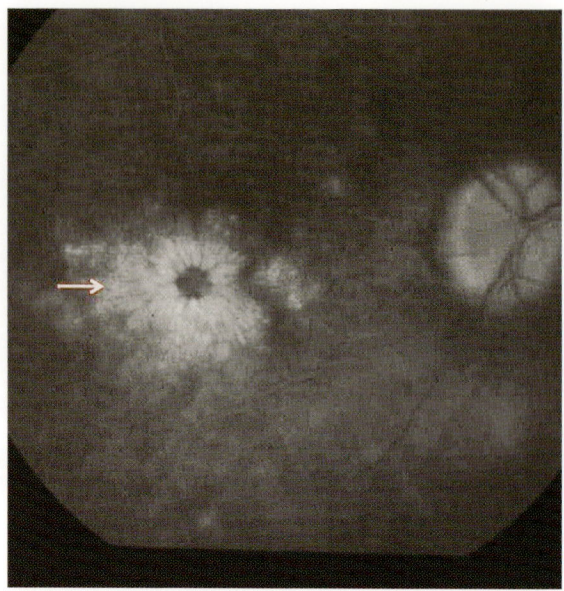

Fig. 3.16. FFA showing late hyperfluorescence (at 6 min) in a "petalloid" pattern. This is characteristic of cystoid macular oedema.

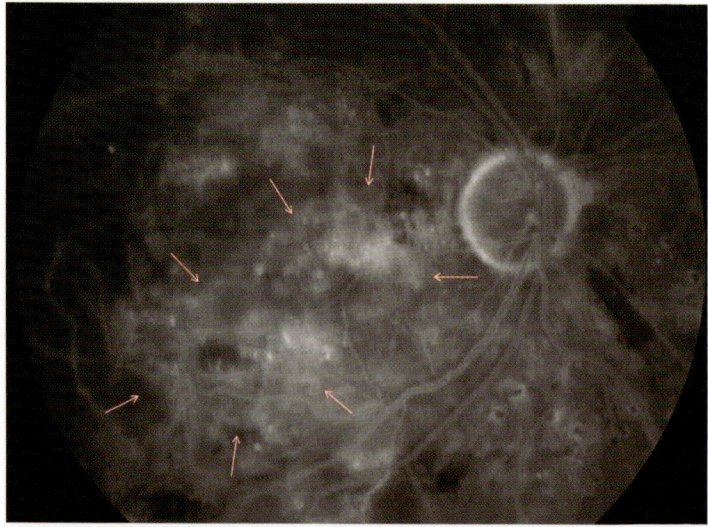

Fig. 3.17. FFA late phase (approximately 6 min) showing diffuse hyperfluorescence in a diabetic patient. This is indicative of diabetic macular oedema (area within red arrows).

RPE which does not change in size and intensity in the late stage (Figs. 3.9, 3.10, 3.11 and 3.12).
- Staining refers to deposition of fluorescein dye within the involved tissue and occurs in both normal and pathological states. Normal structures such as the optic disc and sclera may stain. Pathological changes such as drusen and disciform scars can also show staining (Figs. 3.18 and 3.19).

Areas of hypofluorescence are seen in the following situations:

- Blockage or masking can be seen due to bleeding within the retina. The major retinal vessels run within the nerve fibre layer, whilst the smaller capillaries run in the inner nuclear layer. Thus, a retinal haemorrhage within the nerve fibre layer will block fluorescence from all the retinal blood vessels, whilst one deeper in the retina will block only the capillary fluorescence (Figs. 3.20 and 3.21).
- Vascular filling defects are defined as areas of decreased blood supply which may be seen in conditions like diabetes and arterial occlusions.

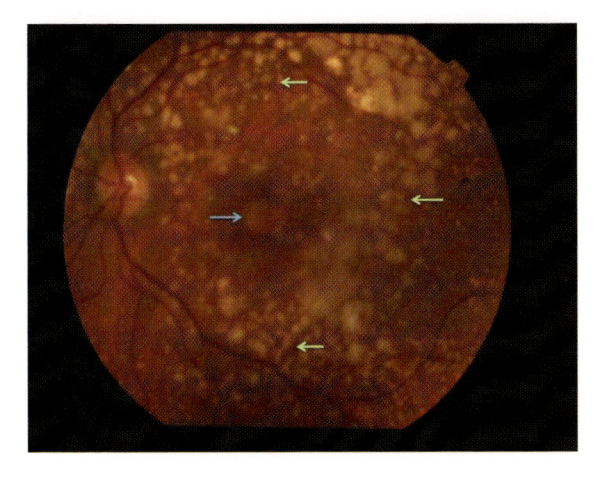

Fig. 3.18. A colour fundus photograph showing central area of RPE atrophy (blue arrow) with numerous scattered drusen (green arrows).

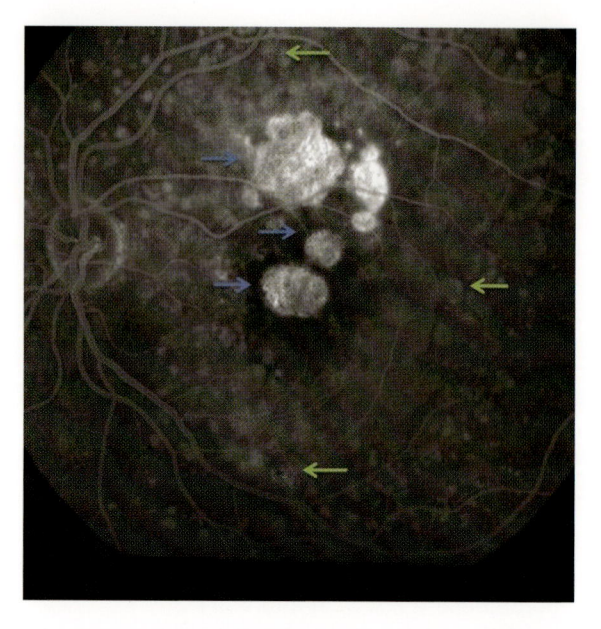

Fig. 3.19. FFA late phase (3 min) of the same eye demonstrating a window defect (blue arrows) alongside staining of drusen (green arrows).

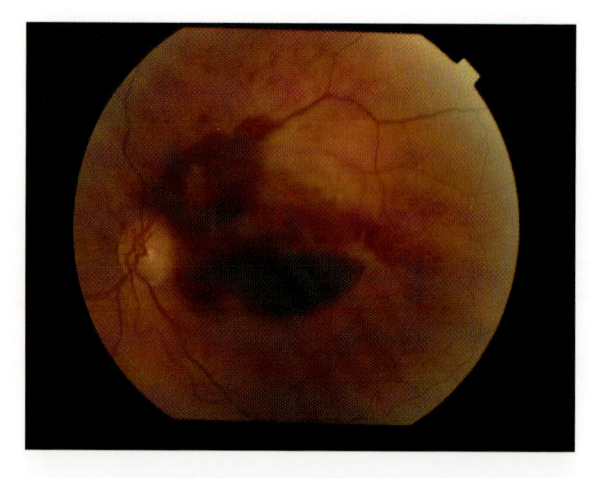

Fig. 3.20. A retinal haemorrhage.

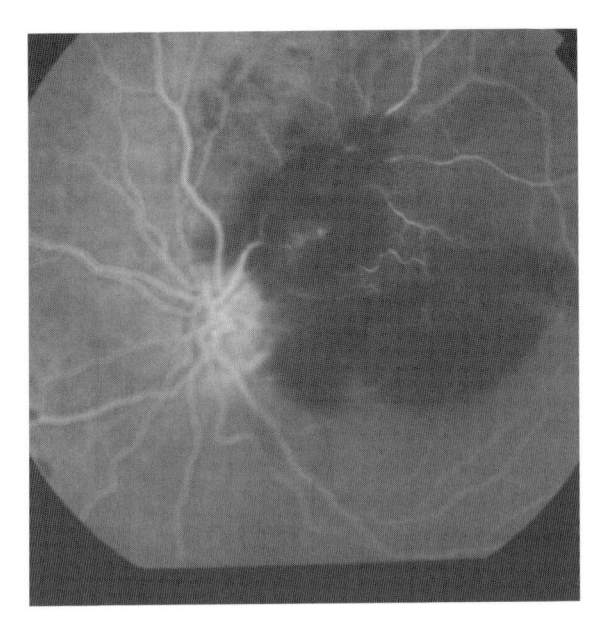

Fig. 3.21. Corresponding FFA showing masking of fluorescence both from retinal and choroidal vasculature in area of haemorrhage.

Points to remember

1. There is no evidence of increased incidence of anaphylaxis to fluorescein in patients with history of anaphylaxis to other drugs or atopy.
2. There is no reported correlation between old age and incidence of adverse reactions (the oldest reported FFA is in a 98-year-old patient).
3. FFA is safe in patients on multiple drugs with no reported adverse reactions due to drug interactions.
4. Hepatic and renal failures are not contraindications to FFA. This is because in such circumstances, plasma half-life of a given dose of fluorescein is prolonged but the peak levels stay the same. Since fluorescein is given only once, there is no risk of cumulative drug toxicity.

(Continued)

> *(Continued)*
> 5. There are no reports of damage to the pregnant woman or foetus with fluorescein. However, pregnancy is a relative contraindication and FFA should be avoided unless absolutely necessary, particularly in the first trimester.
> 6. Fluorescein is excreted for up to 4 days in breast milk. Thus, breast feeding should be avoided for this duration. During this time the women should use a breast pump and discard the milk.
> 7. There is no evidence of increased incidence of serious adverse events with uncontrolled diabetes or hypertension.

> ## Further reading
>
> We would recommend the following article which we have referenced from as well:
>
> *Fluorescein angiography: safety issues and misconceptions* by Sanjay Mishra, Dania Al-Nuaimi, Rita Mclauchlan and Sajjad Mahmood. Published in Eye News, Dec/Jan 2013.

4

THE TECHNIQUE

The following is based on published guidance to reflect the latest clinical practice. There may be minor interdepartmental variations although the general principles remain the same.

> ## ONE STOP AND TWO STOP CLINICS
>
> It is important to emphasise here that the technique described below is for a "one-stop" clinic where the clinician reviews the patient and the injection is delivered by a nurse practitioner straight away. In this scenario, the pre-injection checks outlined in Appendix A will already have been done by the clinician and the nurse practitioner will simply have to fill in the section relating to the actual injecting process itself (please remember that the allergy, consent and correct eye marked should be checked again by the nurse practitioner). In contrast, a "two-stop" process is where the patient is seen by a clinician and a decision made to treat. The patient is then booked onto a separate injecting list usually within a week or two for the nurse practitioner to inject. In this scenario, the pre-injection checks have to be repeated by the practitioner on the day and so familiarity with how to do these is important. In the second scenario, it is also important for the nurse practitioner to make sure a clinician responsible for the list is accessible in case a complication occurs.

1. Confirm the identity of the patient with their notes (including name and date of birth). Do not proceed if the patient's notes are not available.
2. Confirm that the patient has signed a consent form and that he/she is able to confirm the eye that is to be treated. It is also essential to make sure the eye to be injected has been marked by the clinician who saw the patient (Fig. 4.1). Do not proceed if the consent form has not been completed or if there is confusion over which eye is to be treated.

NEAR MISS SCENARIOS

A few examples are worth remembering.

Two patients with the same name were in the waiting area. When the name was called, the wrong patient walked in but because of the appropriate checks the error was picked up instantly and no harm was done.

A clinician forgot to mark the eye to be injected in clinic. This led to some confusion and the nurse practitioner was about to inject the wrong eye. Thankfully, the patient pointed the error out and no harm was done.

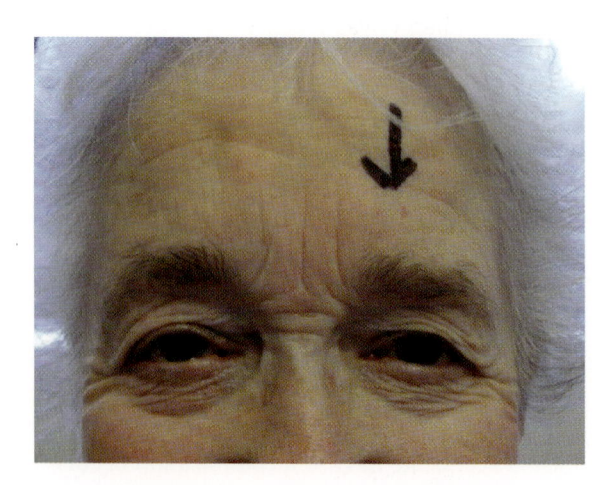

Fig. 4.1. Correct eye marked.

3. Instill topical anaesthesia with proxymetacaine and tetracaine (Fig. 4.2), followed by 5% povidone-iodine into the inferior fornix (Fig. 4.3). Instill proxymetacaine first as this does not sting. It is very important to flood the eye (conjunctival sac) with iodine (do not simply just clean the lids), since the commensal bacteria on the conjunctiva must be exposed to the iodine in order to kill them. Endophthalmitis following intravitreal injection is the most feared complication, and the risk can be substantially reduced with strict attention to the preparation of the injection site.

Note it is important to confirm whether or not the patient has any allergies prior to using iodine. If they are allergic to iodine then an alternative aseptic solution must be used (usually aqueous chlorhexidine).

CRITICAL INCIDENT

A patient developed a localised allergic reaction (swollen lid with itching) due to iodine use. This was documented but iodine was inadvertently applied the next time as well. Thankfully, the allergy was localised and the patient recovered without any long term sequelae. As an injecting list can be very busy, this case highlights the need to double check allergies (to iodine and to any antibiotics) both with the patient and in the notes — "first do no harm."

---

4. Practitioner to wash hands and use sterile gloves (hat and mask must be worn).
5. Set up the injecting kit (Fig. 4.4). For Lucentis® withdraw 0.2 mL through a large blunt filter needle into 1 mL syringe; place a 30 gauge precision glide needle and expel excess without drawing back so 0.05 mL (which for Lucentis® is equivalent to 0.5 mg) remains for injection. Avastin® and

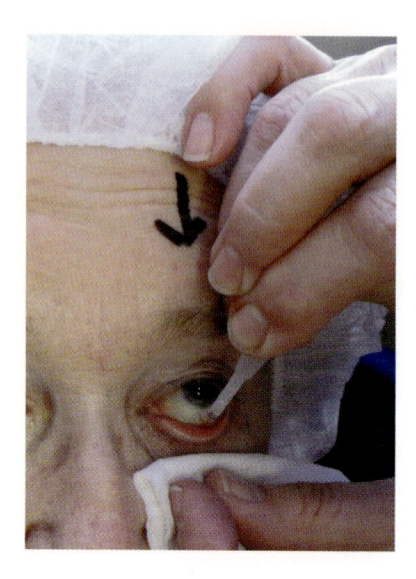

Fig. 4.2. Topical anaesthesia. Pulling the lower lid down exposes the inferior fornix and the drops can be delivered here. When the patient blinks, they are distributed over the anterior surface of the eye.

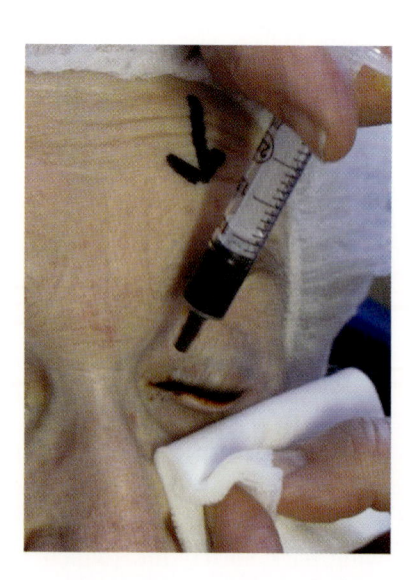

Fig. 4.3. 5% povidone-iodine to inferior fornix.

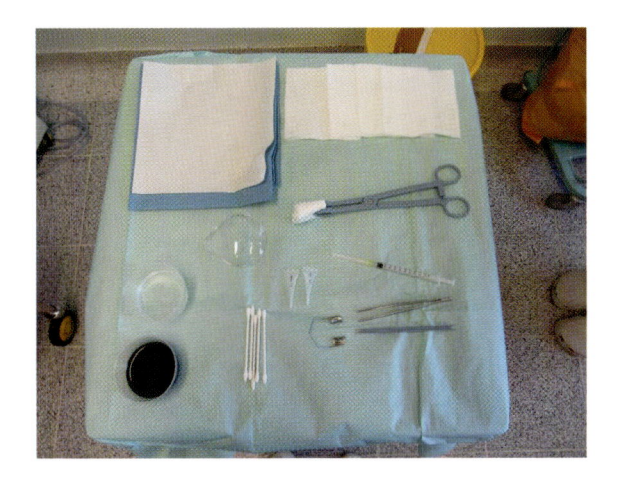

Fig. 4.4. Injection pack.

Eylea® come preloaded in injecting syringes so simply attach aforementioned 30 gauge needle and expel excess until 0.05 mL (which is equivalent to 1.25 mg for Avastin® and 2.0 mg for Eylea) remains for injection. For all other intravitreal injections, the principle remains the same but it is important to make sure the appropriate dose is being given.

6. Apply full iodine preparation (10% povidone-iodine skin preparation) to the lids and surrounding skin prior to draping (Fig. 4.5). Remember that 5% povidone-iodine should already have been applied to the conjunctival sac and been left for 3 min to ensure eradication of all conjunctival bacterial flora (as described in step 3).This is a vital step to reduce the risk of endophthalmitis. If this has not already been done, then ensure it is completed before proceeding any further.
7. Apply sterile drape and sterile speculum (Figs. 4.6 and 4.7).
8. Ask the patient to look into the corner opposite to where you plan to inject. For example, if planning to inject in the superotemporal quadrant, ask the patient to look down and in (inferonasally). In the quadrant where you plan to inject, measure the pars planar injection site 4 mm back from the limbus in phakic eyes (eyes that have their natural lens and

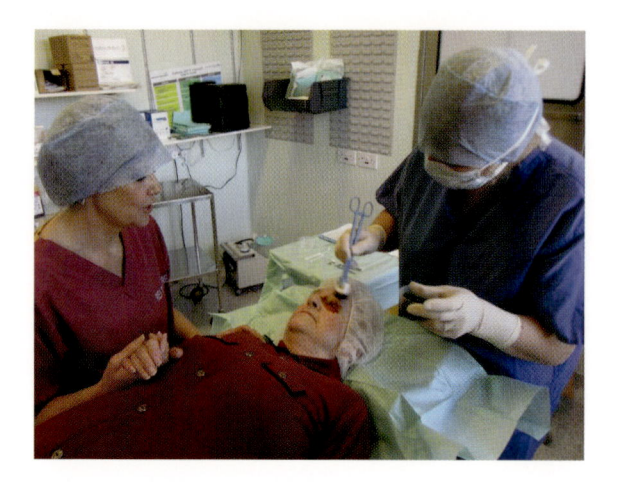

Fig. 4.5. 10% povidone-iodine prep prior to draping.

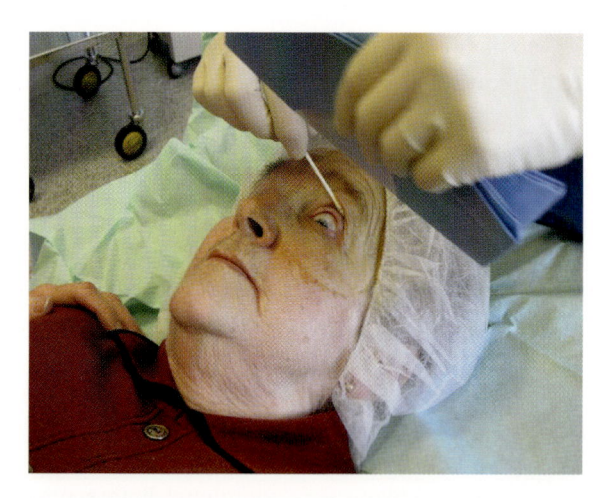

Fig. 4.6. Correct drape technique — ask patient to look to their feet whilst exerting traction on the upper lid. This will allow the drape to engage the upper lid lashes and avoid contact with the injecting needle.

have not had cataract surgery) or 3.5 mm back from the limbus in aphakic/pseudophakic eyes (those that have no lens or have had cataract surgery and now have an artificial intraocular lens).

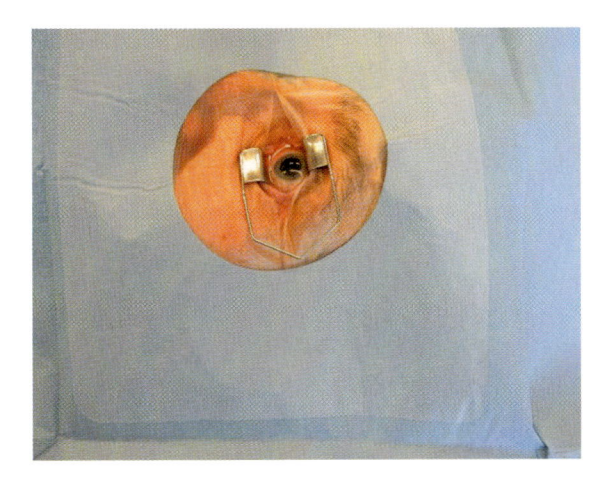

Fig. 4.7. Drape and sterile speculum correctly in place.

Angle the needle posteriorly and aim so that the needle is perpendicular (at right angle) to the surface of the eye whilst also directed towards the central core of the vitreous. Using the correct entry point and correct angle will ensure that the needle passes safely through the pars plana and into the vitreous cavity without damaging the lens or the retina. If the needle is too close to the limbus or if the needle is angled too close to the lens, then it will touch the lens and cause a traumatic cataract. If the needle is too far away from the limbus, then the needle will pass through the retina and cause a retinal tear and retinal detachment. Also avoid contact with the lid margin (to reduce contamination of the needle with any possible bacteria). The bevel of the needle should be facing upwards. Sliding the conjunctiva circumferentially so the scleral entry point does not coincide with the conjunctival entry point is advisable (so after the injection has been completed, the conjunctiva will slide back and the hole in the conjunctiva will not lie directly over the hole in the sclera, theoretically reducing the risk of bacterial infection subsequently entering the eye).

9. Avoid three o'clock and nine o'clock injection sites as the long ciliary nerves run in this position and can cause pain

despite adequate topical anaesthesia. Also consider rotating quadrants when repeated injections are going to be needed since thinning of the sclera can result from multiple injections. Some patients have pre-existing areas of scleral thinning which give a brownish hue due to the visible underlying choroid. These should be avoided. Instill further anaesthetic drops (proxymetacaine or tetracaine) to the quadrant to be injected.

10. Sterile calliper should be used to measure the injection distance (Fig. 4.8).
11. Use a 30-gauge needle no longer than 15 mm to inject. 1/2-to 2/3rds of the needle is advanced into the eye (Fig. 4.9).
12. Inject the drug slowly over a few seconds. Then wait a few seconds more before removing the needle in a single, controlled movement. This pause helps reduce the risk of drug reflux out of the injection site.
13. After the needle is removed, a sterile cotton bud (soaked in povidone-iodine) should be applied to the entry site for 10 sec.
14. The injection site should be wiped radially away from the limbus to remove any vitreous wick.

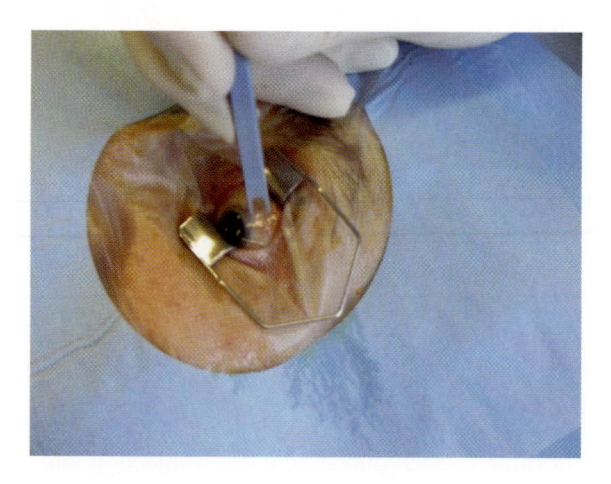

Fig. 4.8. Calliper to measure distance from the limbus.

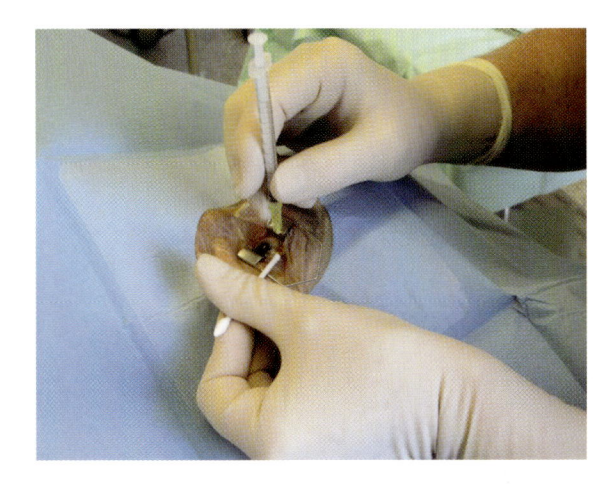

Fig. 4.9. Injection being delivered into the superotemporal quadrant.

15. Apply topical antibiotics to the cornea and injection site.
16. Check to see if the patient can see counting fingers at 1 m using the injected eye (by covering the other eye).
17. Some departments have a policy requiring the placement of an eye shield over the injected eye.
18. Some patients may be asked to have their intraocular pressures measured by the clinician post injection.
19. Ensure the patient has a prescription for antibiotics based on departmental preference. Remember to check for allergies to antibiotics.
20. Complete the intraocular procedure component of the patient pathway and ensure the patient's name has been included in the intravitreal injection logbook. This is usually an A4 sized diary in which the patients' details, date of the injection, name of medicine injected, eye injected and name of injector is documented.

Remember to document that the patient could see counting fingers with the injected eye post treatment. In the event that a patient cannot see counting fingers with the treated eye, the patient must be taken immediately to the clinician responsible, to consider whether intervention is required. The concern is

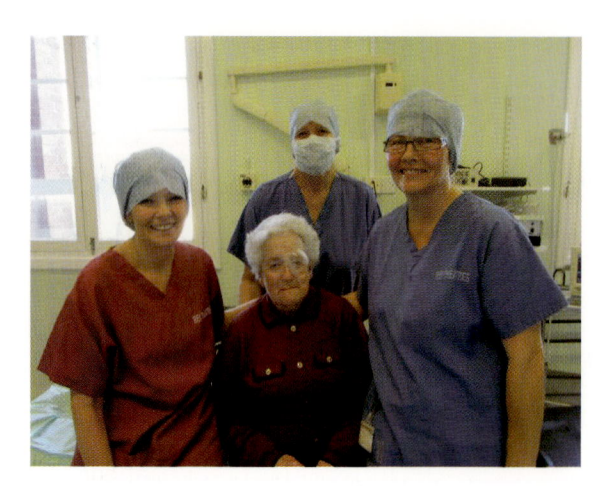

Fig. 4.10. A comfortable patient and satisfied team at the end (Royal Eye Infirmary, Plymouth).

that the intravitreal injection may have raised the intraocular pressure to a high level causing a central retinal artery occlusion. The clinician may decide to release fluid from the peripheral cornea using an insulin syringe, MVR blade or paracentesis blade resulting in a rapid reduction in intraocular pressure and restoration of central retinal artery blood flow. Time is critical here and it is wise to always ensure that the responsible clinician know that you are still injecting so that they remain easily accessible. Also it is sensible to check before every list, where the required instruments are so that valuable time is not lost searching for them.

Important points to remember

The following concepts will help in ensuring a competent intravitreal injection.

(a) **Effect of positioning of the eye**
Ask the patient to look away from the quadrant you wish to inject and imagine where the centre of the eye is in relation to the injection point. If you enter perpendicular to the sclera here, the 15 mm needle cannot reach the opposite retina.

(b) Positioning of the needle in relation to ocular structures
Any forward tilt of the needle will run the risk of lens damage. Backward or sideways tilt can be safe as long as the needle does not go in completely. An oblique entry like this may theoretically reduce vitreous loss and the resulting longer track may also reduce the risk of bacteria entering the eye.

(c) Thoroughness about checking the correct patient and the correct eye. Injection lists are typically busy so there is a real danger of human error resulting in the incorrect patient/incorrect eye being injected.

(d) Care to ensure the injection site is prepared meticulously with povidone-iodine to reduce the risk of endophthalmitis. Remember of course that patients with ocular surface infections (such as conjunctivitis, microbial keratitis), uncontrolled blepharitis or nasolacrimal duct obstruction should not have intravitreal injections since this will increase their risk of endophthalmitis. Therefore, if your patient has a red, irritable or watery eye prior to treatment then you should not proceed until this is first addressed.

(e) Other pitfalls: pathology in some quadrants may make the procedure more dangerous, e.g. tumours or previous retinal detachment surgery (which has involved buckles or bands placed around the eye).

5

COMPLICATIONS

The reason why patients give their informed consent for an intravitreal injection is because, on balance, they perceive that the potential benefits of treatment outweigh the risks.

As with any surgical procedure there is potential for complications at any stage and it is important for the practitioner to be aware of these.

WRONG PATIENT OR WRONG EYE INJECTED

There is a rapid turnover of patients receiving this treatment, so extra care is needed to ensure that the correct patient has the correct eye treated. All patients should have a mark over the eye to be injected. If both eyes are to be injected, then a mark over both is mandatory. Always confirm with the patient his/her name, date of birth and eye to be injected prior to proceeding.

IODINE USED IN A PATIENT WITH IODINE ALLERGY

Before instilling eye drops and cleaning with povidone-iodine, ask the patient if he/she has any allergies AND cross-check this in the notes. Specifically ask if the patient had an iodine allergy in the past. Swelling of the lid, redness of the eye and excessive discomfort should raise concern of a localised allergy and a doctor should be informed immediately. If the patient becomes systemically unwell (short of breath, collapse and rash), then follow the hospitals' guideline for anaphylaxis.

PATIENT COLLAPSE

This may be due to the stress of the procedure exacerbating a patient's underlying medical condition (severe heart or lung disease). If a patient appears particularly unwell, then check with a doctor to see if the procedure is still necessary. Alternatively, collapse may be due to anaphylaxis to the iodine or intravitreal agent, in which case you should follow the hospitals' guidelines on anaphylaxis.

For any patient who collapses, call for help. Check for signs of life (pulse, breathing, movement). If there are no signs of life, immediately call the cardiac arrest team (dial 2222 — do NOT go through switch as this takes too long) and begin basic life support (chest compressions and ventilations) until those able to provide advanced life support arrive.

SUBCONJUNCTIVAL HAEMORRHAGE

This is a common but relatively minor complication, which occurs since the intravitreal injection needle must pass through the conjunctiva (Fig. 5.1). Patients on anti-platelet or anti-coagulation medication are at particular risk. If this occurs, explain to the patient that it should resolve in a week or so.

PROBLEMS ASSOCIATED WITH A DILATED PUPIL

In some susceptible individuals, dilating a pupil can cause the intraocular pressure to rapidly rise ("acute glaucoma"). This is

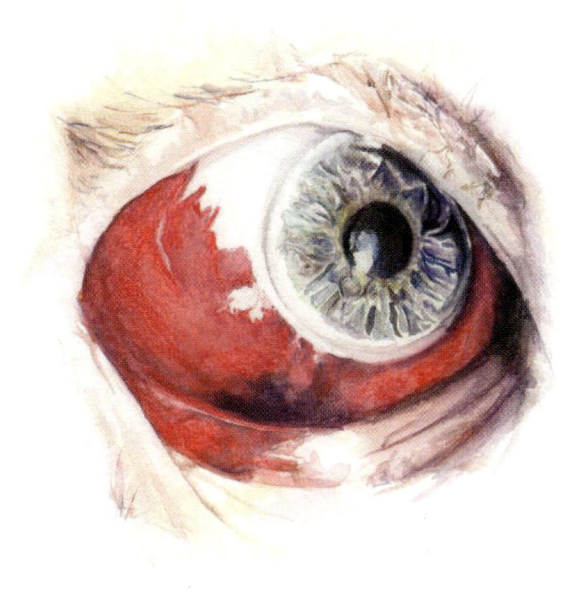

Fig. 5.1. Subconjunctival haemorrhage.

more common in hypermetropes (long sighted) and the elderly, especially if there is a concurrent nuclear sclerotic cataract.

This risk is rare and if there is concern, this should be discussed with an ophthalmologist prior to dilating the pupil. There is no risk to patients with open angle glaucoma (the more common form of glaucoma) and the risk is only present for patients with narrow anterior chamber angles. However, eye clinic personnel need to be aware of this risk, so if a patient reports pain or significantly blurred vision following the instillation of mydriatics, their eye pressure should be checked and a doctor informed.

Some elderly patients may have had cataract surgery in the past with a "lobster claw iris clip" intraocular lens implant (Fig. 5.2). These patients should not be dilated. The patient will usually be aware of this and not let anybody dilate their eyes. Patients with artisan-style iris claw lenses can usually be safely dilated.

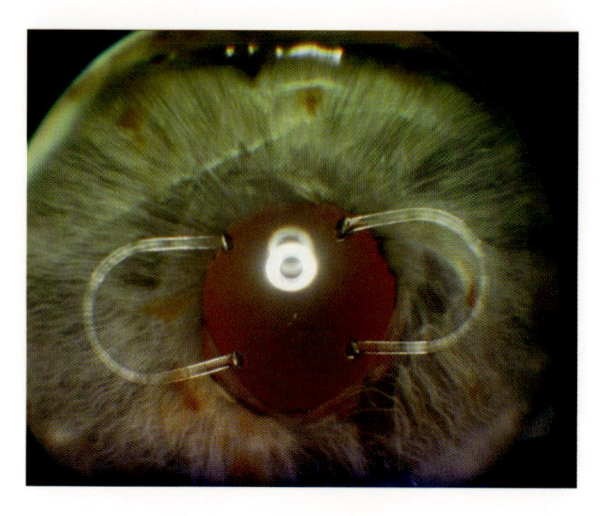

Fig. 5.2. A "lobster claw iris clip" lens. This was placed in patients with no capsular support to stabilise the lens (e.g. after intracapsular cataract extraction). Dilation of the pupil may unhinge the clips causing the lens to fall into the back of the eye (photo courtesy of Mr. Peter Simcock).

CORNEAL ABRASION

The cornea can be traumatised by the insertion of the speculum or a wayward needle. If the cornea is damaged (Fig. 5.3), then inform a doctor who can assess further and consider additional treatment or altered follow-up.

TOXIC EPITHELIOPATHY OF CORNEA

This occurs if excessive povidone-iodine or local anaesthetic affects the cornea, which is why we use lower strength iodine. Always irrigate both the injection site and cornea with a topical antibiotic after the procedure. Avoid priming syringes over the cornea.

CATARACT

If the intravitreal injection needle enters the eye too anteriorly or is angled too anteriorly, then the lens can be damaged. This

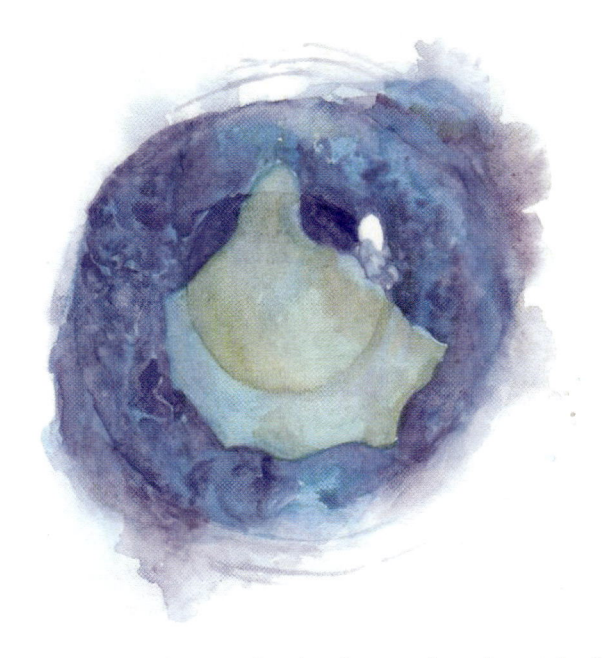

Fig. 5.3. Corneal abrasion showing fluorescein stain uptake (yellow green area) when viewed using a blue filter on a slit lamp.

will result in a traumatic cataract and the patient may require subsequent cataract surgery. Traumatic cataracts such as these can become manifest very quickly (same day) and surgically are complex to treat since the lens capsule will also be damaged. Managing traumatic cataracts is therefore more complicated and challenging than age-related cataracts. For this reason it is important to be careful and always avoid lens contact with your needle.

POSTERIOR VITREOUS DETACHMENT AND RETINAL TEARS/DETACHMENT

An intravitreal injection can cause the posterior lining of the vitreous to detach from the retina. This, in itself, is usually harmless although the patient may notice more floaters. However, this process can also cause a retinal tear. Furthermore,

46 ♦ *Intravitreal Injections*

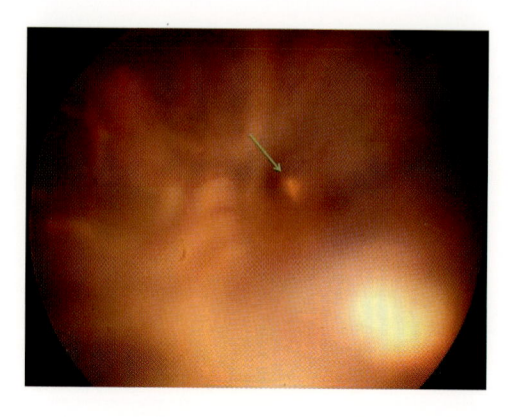

Fig. 5.4. Complete retinal detachment. Note that the retinal details are not clear and it looks elevated. The optic disc is barely visible (arrow). (Photo courtesy of Dr. Nalinda Samrakoon, Royal Eye Infirmary, Plymouth.)

if the intravitreal needle enters the eye too posteriorly or is angled too posteriorly then the retina can be torn. Failure to detect and treat a retinal tear can result in the development of a retinal detachment (neurosensory retina peels off from the RPE), which causes permanent loss of vision if not detected and treated promptly.

RAISED INTRAOCULAR PRESSURE (IOP)/CENTRAL RETINAL ARTERY OCCLUSION/ISCHEMIC OPTIC NEUROPATHY

If this occurs, it is usually transient and mild. However, if the patient has glaucoma or ocular hypertension, it may be necessary to check the IOP both before and after treatment the same day. In consultation with a doctor, appropriate plans to check IOP should be made.

Rarely, the IOP can rise rapidly to very high levels. This can damage the retina (by causing a central retinal artery occlusion) or the optic nerve (ischaemic optic neuropathy). For this reason, it is important to routinely check that the patient can see fingers (counting fingers acuity) after the intravitreal injection. If the patient can do this, then such a high rise in IOP is unlikely. If a

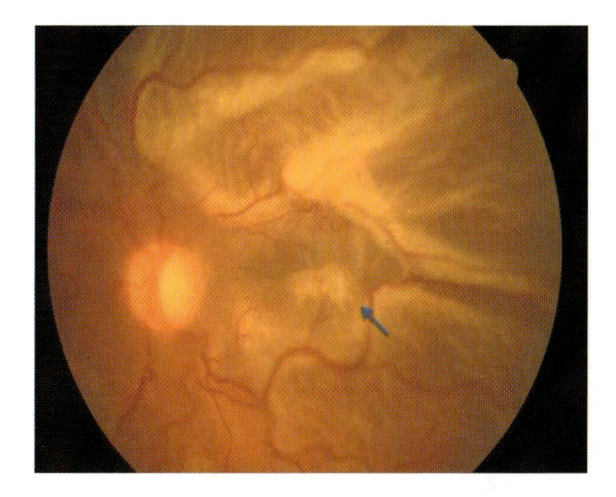

Fig. 5.5. A partial retinal detachment in the left eye (macula off). Note that the macula appears elevated with folds due to underlying subretinal fluid (blue arrow). The optic disc and nasal retina appears intact. (Photo courtesy of Mr. Peter Simcock.)

patient cannot see counting fingers after an intravitreal injection, then a doctor must be informed immediately and anterior chamber paracentesis considered.

AIR BUBBLES

When the drug is injected into the vitreous, there is a chance that air will also be injected inadvertently (usually trapped in the needle). This can cause more floaters than normal but the problem usually resolves within a couple of days. If there is a concern that a large amount of air has entered the vitreous, then the intraocular pressure should be checked and the problem discussed with a doctor.

VITREOUS WICKS

When the intravitreal needle is removed, sometimes vitreous may herniate through the scleral wound. This vitreous wick can act as a pathway for conjunctival bacteria to gain access into the vitreous cavity and cause endophthalmitis. Wait for a few seconds after the injection is complete, to reduce reflux of the drug, and remove the needle slowly. Put pressure on the injection site for 10 sec to reduce secondary vitreous loss. This complication can also be reduced by displacing the conjunctiva to one side before injecting, thus ensuring that the conjunctival entry point does not overlie the scleral entry point. Ten percent of injections are thought to leave some vitreous on the surface, which is why it is important to always use a sterile cotton tip and wipe away from the limbus over the injection site (once the needle is withdrawn).

ENDOPHTHALMITIS

This is perhaps the most devastating complication that can occur with intravitreal injections (Figs. 5.6 and 5.7). Endophthalmitis refers to a severe, sight threatening eye infection involving the vitreous cavity and anterior chamber. In addition to causing

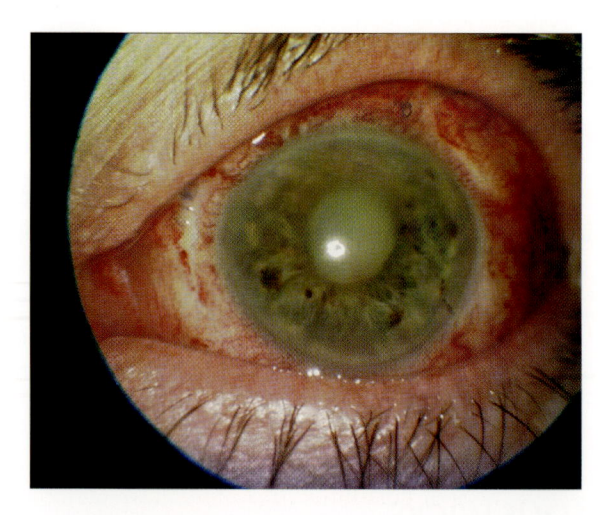

Fig. 5.6. Endophthalmitis. Note that the eye is inflamed with an absent red reflex. Hypopyon (pus in the anterior chamber) is commonly seen but is absent in this eye.

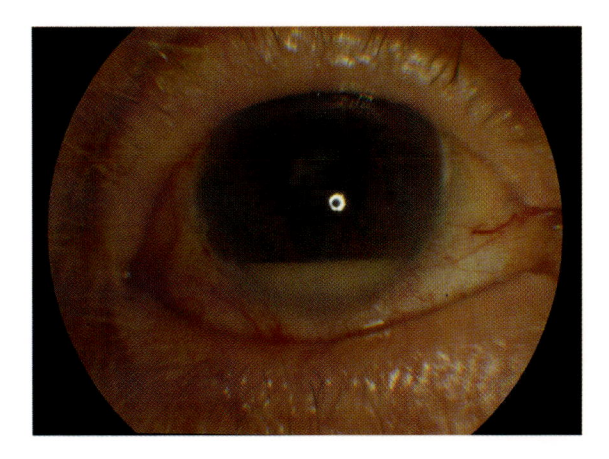

Fig. 5.7. An eye with endophthalmitis. Note the presence of pus in the anterior chamber (hypopyon). (Photo courtesy of Mr. Peter Simcock.)

visual loss, severe cases unresponsive to treatment may require the eye to be eviscerated.

By ensuring adherence to a strict aseptic technique and appropriate storage of intravitreal agents, this risk is minimised to approximately 1 in 1,000 per injection. Patients should be aware of this risk and advised to contact the eye department immediately should they experience increasing eye pain, redness or deterioration in vision.

IMPORTANT STUDY

Post Intravitreal Anti-VEGF Endophthalmitis in the United Kingdom: Incidence, Features, Risk Factors and Outcomes

This was a prospective observational case control study performed by the British Ophthalmic Surveillance Unit (BOSU). Forty-seven cases of post-intravitreal anti-VEGF endophthal-

(*Continued*)

(Continued)

mitis (PIAE) were identified between January 2009 and March 2010 throughout the UK. Thus, the estimated incidence of PIAE was found to be 0.025%. Mean age of presentation was 78 years. Mean number of injections before PIAE was 5. Mean days to presentation was 5 (range 1–39). Positive microbiology cultures were obtained in 59.6% of cases, giving a culture positive incidence of 0.015%. The majority of causative organisms were gram positive (92.8%). The most common presenting symptom was reduction in vision (96%), followed by pain/photophobia and redness. The most common signs were vitritis, hyperaemia and hypopyon. The majority of patients (63.6%) had worse vision after 6 months follow-up when compared with acuity pre-PIAE.

Significant risk factors were:

1. Failure to administer topical antibiotic drops immediately after injection.
2. Blepharitis.
3. Subconjunctival anaesthesia.
4. Patient squeezing during injection.
5. Failure to administer topical antibiotics before anti-VEGF injection.

Recommendations made were:

1. Adequate treatment of blepharitis and eyelid check before injecting.
2. Avoidance of subconjunctival anaesthesia if possible.
3. Administration of topical antibiotics immediately after injection.
4. To consider administering topical antibiotics before the injection. This step was left to the discretion of the clinician.

The citation for the full paper is:

DAM lyall *et al.* (2012) Post-intravitreal anti-VEGF endophthalmitis in the United Kingdom: incidence, features, risk factors and outcomes. *Eye* **26**: 1517–1526.

IMPORTANT: Please remember that most practitioners are very cautious as they start doing intravitreal injections. However, as experience is gained there is a risk of going into "auto-pilot" mode, especially on high volume lists which may result in not every step being given appropriate attention, thus leading to complications. It is important to remember that each eye being injected is precious and only by giving every step of every injection due attention can complications be minimised.

Further reading

The following paper presents a good review of ocular and systemic complications associated with intravitreal anti-VEGF agents:

- Falavarjani KG, Nguyen QD. (2013) Adverse events and complications associated with intravitreal injection of anti-VEGF agents: a review of literature. *Eye* **27**: 787–794.

6

PROTOTYPE TRAINING STRUCTURE

Proceeding with a specialised role can often be a daunting decision for nurses to make. However, once the decision has been made there may be further challenges ahead. In areas where nurses have only recently started to take on extended roles, training structures can be lacking. Intravitreal injection training at present has no defined curriculum either by the Royal College of Nursing or the Royal College of Ophthalmologists. It is thus left to the individual departments to try and forge a training structure and this can be time consuming. Here, we outline a scheme we have used in our region over the last few years. The readers can feel free to adopt it in its entirety or modify it to suit their departmental needs. In our experience, both trainers and trainees have found it relevant and easy to undertake.

1) REQUIREMENTS OF STAFF PERFORMING INTRAVITREAL INJECTIONS

1. Must be a registered Ophthalmic Nurse, Optometrist or Orthoptist.
2. Hold the ENB 346 course (Ophthalmic Nursing) or equivalent orthoptic or optometric experience with a minimum of 1 year's consolidation.

3. Have a reasonable level of stereopsis.
4. Be experienced in other procedures that ensure the individual has a degree of manual dexterity (e.g. Sub-tenon's injections, botulinum toxin injections, incision and curettage of chalazia, electrolysis). Staff will also have to perform supervised "mock" intravitreal injections on pig eyes.
5. Receive two tutorials from ophthalmic medical staff.
6. Review the basic knowledge in this handbook. All practitioners will be required to demonstrate background knowledge by obtaining at least 80% marks in a MCQ examination.
7. Complete a 3-month training programme with a consultant ophthalmologist and obtain certificate of accreditation.
8. Be observed performing 10 intravitreal injections by a second consultant ophthalmologist.

2) REASSESSMENT

Staff will require reassessment every year by a consultant ophthalmologist (3 observed injections) at which point they will also have to produce evidence of ongoing learning, self assessment and log book. If there is a lapse of clinical practice for 12 weeks or more, then reassessment by a consultant will also be required.

3) CLINICAL GOVERNANCE

The practitioner will keep a diary of all injections undertaken whilst under supervision. For the first 50 cases after accreditation, the consultant responsible will assess the patient one month later to check for complications. Outcomes will be reported in the diary.

During this period, a protocol used for pain assessment will be used to feedback patient satisfaction. Results will then be compared with a previous baseline audit of consultant practice.

A log of all injections will be kept as evidence for annual reassessments.

4) TRAINING PROGRAMME

The practitioner will be expected to read this handbook.

This basic knowledge will be reinforced with two 1-hour tutorials describing the intravitreal injection technique by a consultant ophthalmologist.

There will be a Multiple Choice Questionnaire (20 key questions) in which the practitioner will have to score 80% correct (no negative marking).

The practitioner will then obtain the following practical experience:

1. The practitioner will observe 20 injections undertaken by a consultant ophthalmologist.
2. The practitioner will then perform 40 intravitreal injections supervised by a consultant ophthalmologist.
3. For these 40 cases, the clinician will examine the patient 10 min after the injection to ensure there has been no immediate complication.
4. If satisfactory, the practitioner will then perform unsupervised injections in the next 20 cases. These patients will also be examined by the clinician 10 min after the procedure to ensure there has been no immediate complication.

There will be a final session once the practical sessions are completed to establish an audit process and patient satisfaction survey.

This training programme should take approximately three months to complete. Once the practitioner has completed this training programme satisfactorily, he/she will then have to inject 10 patients, observed by a second independent clinician to be finally accredited.

5) ACCREDITATION

The following competencies should be assessed at the end of the three-month training period by a second independent clinician for accreditation:

1. Preparation and maintenance of the intravitreal injection room.
2. Understanding of the consenting process.
3. Understanding of the role of a supporting Health Care Assistant.
4. Preparation of the patient and monitoring requirements.
5. Intravitreal injection (10 injections observed).
6. Post injection assessment of the patients.
7. Understanding of complications.
8. Management of complications and understanding when and how to call for help.
9. Post injection patient instructions.
10. Procedure for responding to a patient collapse.

6) GUIDELINES FOR ASSESSORS

When undertaking instruction and assessment and before signing the certificate of competence, assessors should satisfy themselves that the practitioners understand:

1. The anatomy of the eye and the orbit.
2. The issues of informed consent.
3. Preparation required, complications and how they are managed alongside the aftercare of a patient.
4. Managing a collapsed patient.
5. The appropriate documentation.
6. Audit and patient satisfaction survey procedures.

IMPORTANT: Please ensure both your trust and the Royal College of Nursing are happy with the medico-legal aspect of injecting. Needless to say, this is important on the rare occasion a complication results in a legal challenge. Your directorate manger can help clarify if trust indemnity covers you for intravitreal injections and you can contact the Royal College of Nursing yourself for clarification.

OUR EXPERIENCE:

A safety audit of the first 10,000 intravitreal Ranibizumab® injections performed by ophthalmic nurse practitioners.

A recent prospective safety audit in our region found that carefully selected and well-trained nurse practitioners are capable of delivering a safe, effective intravitreal injection treatment service. Two trained nurse practitioners administered 10,006 injections in the first 5.5 years of the service (1st May 2008 to 8th October 2013). This represented 84.1% of the total injections performed within the unit during this period. Four patients developed presumed infectious endophthalmitis (one was culture-positive and three were culture negative). The incidence of post-injection endophthalmitis was therefore 0.04%, which compares favourably to the rate established by the British Ophthalmic Surveillance Unit. There was no evidence of lens touch, retinal detachment or systemic thromboembolic events. This work demonstrates how such a service can be established and provides safety data that other units can use as a benchmark when evaluating their own practice.

This study has been submitted for peer review and publication.

7

SETTING UP A WETLAB

Organising a wetlab session can be invaluable for training to do intravitreal injections. This can easily be done by following the steps:

1. Supervised "mock" intravitreal injections on pigs' eyes are performed as per the technique described earlier.
2. Split pig heads (split down the centre as shown in Figs. 7.1 and 7.2) can be easily acquired from your local butcher. We have used these very successfully in local courses for ophthalmologists and to train our nurse practitioners as well.
3. The pigs' heads should be kept in a tray as shown, to avoid spillage of fluids used.
4. The complete procedure can easily be practised, starting from draping all the way through to giving the injection.
5. Special care should be taken to dispose of the anatomical waste (i.e. pigs' heads). Most hospitals require the use of yellow bin bags that have to be placed in special clinical waste collection areas. Please consult your hospitals' clinical waste disposal team for specific instructions.

60 ♦ *Intravitreal Injections*

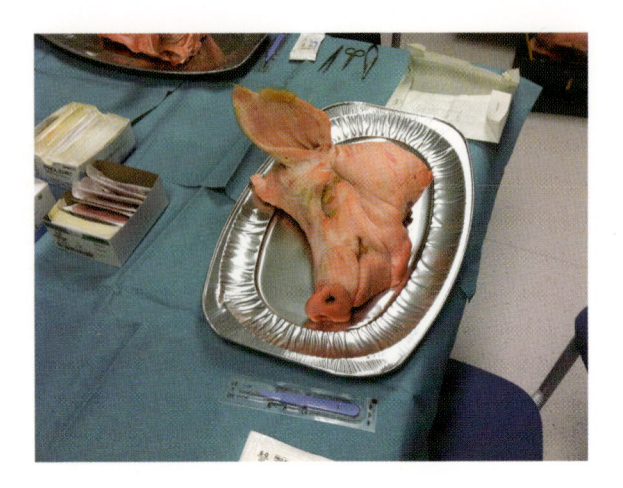

Fig. 7.1. A split pig head.

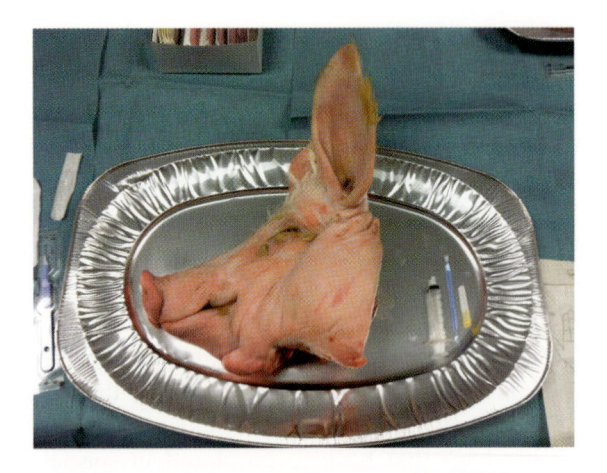

Fig. 7.2. Split pig head with injecting equipment.

8

ORGANISING A DEDICATED CLEAN ROOM

Intravitreal injections may be carried out in a theatre or in a dedicated clean room in outpatients. The volume of injections required on a daily basis in most eye units has led to the vast majority being done in outpatients. Whilst organising a clean room, the following precautions must be kept in mind:

1. It should deal only with non-infected cases and be free from interruptions. Check with your local Infection Control Team regarding the exact specifications of a clean room in your hospital.
2. The room must have good illumination and washable floors (as confirmed by the local Health and Safety regulations).
3. Ceiling should be non-particulate in nature so that no dust or debris can fall onto the operating field.
4. Resuscitation facilities should be available nearby. The room should also have a reclining chair or a bed with an adjustable incline to be able to change the patients' position in case an emergency occurs.

Further information can be found in the following resources:

1. *The Royal College of Ophthalmologists: Guidelines for Intravitreal Injections Procedure 2009.*
2. *Department of Health: Health Building Note 00-09. Infection Control in the Built Environment.* (Published, March 2013.)

FURTHER READING

For further reading we recommend the following excellent textbooks:

Clinical Anatomy of the Eye by Richard S Snell and Michael A Lemp (Blackwell Publishing).

Clinical Ophthalmology: A Systematic Approach by Jack J Kanski (Elsevier Publishing).

APPENDIX A: INTRAVITREAL INJECTION CHECKLIST

> Patient surname:
> First name:
> Hospital Number:
> DOB:
> Affix patient label here if available

PRE-INJECTION ASSESSMENT

- **Allergies (including latex):**
- **Written consent:** Yes/No
- **Recent stroke/TIA:** Yes/No
- **Recent cardiac episode:** Yes/No
- **Current vision:** Rt: Lt:
- **Blepharitis:**
  Present: Treated with:
  Not present:
- **Regurgitation test (check for lacrimal sac collection):**
  Present: Treated with:
  Not present:
- **Correct eye marked:** Yes/No

Record of Procedure

Date:
Right/Left intravitreal (write name of drug):
Performed by: Injection no:
Povidone iodine/Chlorhexidine prep:
Dose of injected drug:
Site of injection:
Can patient count fingers at end:
Complications:
Follow up arrangements:

NOTES TO ASSIST PRE-INJECTION ASSESSMENT

Blepharitis This is a chronic inflammatory condition of the eyelids. It is most commonly caused by a dysfunction of the oily glands in the lids (meibomian glands). This is called seborrheic blepharitis. It can also be caused by a mild bacterial infection (staphylococcal blepharitis) and sometimes the two forms coexist. Commonly seen signs are:

- Flaking, scaling and crusting around the eyelashes like dandruff (Fig. A.1).
- Red eyelids especially around the eyelashes.
- Soreness and irritation.
- In severe cases, small ulcers can develop alongside the eyelashes which can bleed.

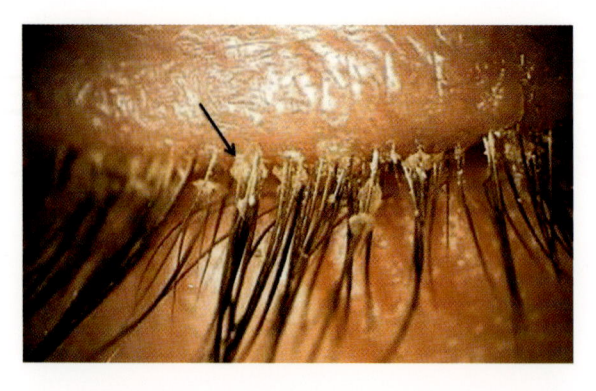

Fig. A.1. Blepharitis with crusting around the eyelashes (arrow).

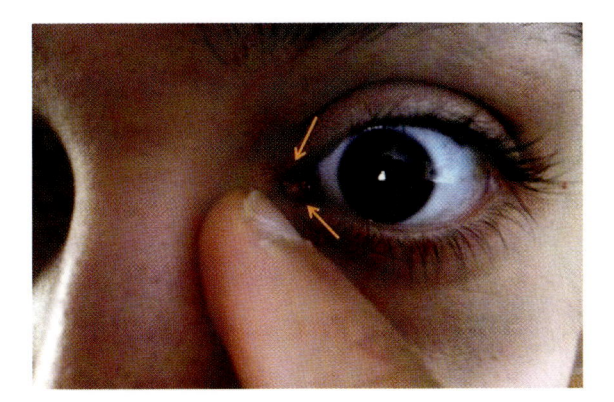

Fig. A.2. Regurgitation test — press on the lacrimal sac with your finger as shown whilst observing the location of the puncta (arrows) for regurgitation.

An eye with blepharitis has a higher chance of developing endophthalmitis after an intravitreal injection therefore it is important to recognise and treat this condition prior to injecting. Usual treatment consists of lid hygiene and antibiotics drops or ointment. The clinician responsible will be able to guide you.

Regurgitation test The lacrimal sac forms part of the lacrimal drainage system of the eyelids. This drains tears from openings in the inner aspect of the eyelids (called the puncta) down into the nose. An obstruction along this system can cause tears to collect in the lacrimal sac with subsequent infection. In the regurgitation test, the lacrimal sac is pressed with a finger (Fig. A.2) whilst the upper and lower puncta are observed with a slit lamp. Regurgitation through the puncta of yellow coloured pus indicates infection and thus a higher chance of endophthalmitis after an intravitreal injection. This must be treated first by a responsible clinician. Treatment would normally include antibiotics to treat infection with subsequent measures to try and resolve the obstruction (usually via a surgical procedure called a dacrocystorhinostomy).

APPENDIX B: BASIC LIFE SUPPORT ALGORITHM

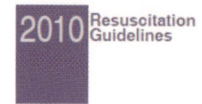

2010 Resuscitation Guidelines

Resuscitation Council (UK)

Adult Basic Life Support

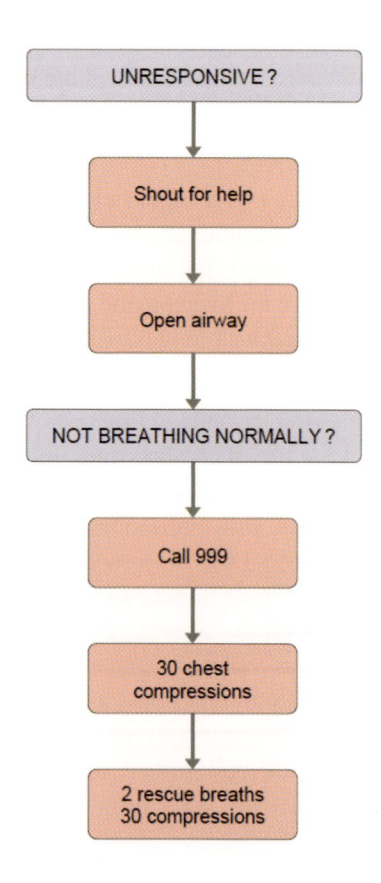

- UNRESPONSIVE?
- Shout for help
- Open airway
- NOT BREATHING NORMALLY?
- Call 999
- 30 chest compressions
- 2 rescue breaths 30 compressions

APPENDIX C: ANAPHYLAXIS ALGORITHM

Resuscitation Council (UK)

Anaphylaxis algorithm

Anaphylactic reaction?

Airway, **B**reathing, **C**irculation, **D**isability, **E**xposure

Diagnosis - look for:
- Acute onset of illness
- Life-threatening Airway and/or Breathing and/or Circulation problems [1]
- And usually skin changes

- **Call for help**
- Lay patient flat
- Raise patient's legs

Adrenaline [2]

When skills and equipment available:
- Establish airway
- High flow oxygen
- IV fluid challenge [3]
- Chlorphenamine [4]
- Hydrocortisone [5]

Monitor:
- Pulse oximetry
- ECG
- Blood pressure

---

[1] **Life-threatening problems:**
Airway: swelling, hoarseness, stridor
Breathing: rapid breathing, wheeze, fatigue, cyanosis, SpO_2 < 92%, confusion
Circulation: pale, clammy, low blood pressure, faintness, drowsy/coma

---

[2] **Adrenaline** *(give IM unless experienced with IV adrenaline)*
IM doses of 1:1,000 adrenaline (repeat after 5 min if no better)
- Adult: 500 micrograms IM (0.5 mL)
- Child more than 12 years: 500 micrograms IM (0.5 mL)
- Child 6 -12 years: 300 micrograms IM (0.3 mL)
- Child less than 6 years: 150 micrograms IM (0.15 mL)

Adrenaline IV to be given **only by experienced specialists**
Titrate: Adults 50 micrograms; Children 1 microgram/kg

[3] **IV fluid challenge:**
Adult - 500 – 1,000 mL
Child - crystalloid 20 mL/kg

Stop IV colloid if this might be the cause of anaphylaxis

---

	4 Chlorphenamine (IM or slow IV)	**5 Hydrocortisone** (IM or slow IV)
Adult or child more than 12 years	10 mg	200 mg
Child 6 - 12 years	5 mg	100 mg
Child 6 months to 6 years	2.5 mg	50 mg
Child less than 6 months	250 micrograms/kg	25 mg

INDEX

abrasion 44, 45
accreditation 54, 55
age-related macular degeneration (AMD) 14
allergy 29, 31, 41, 42
anaesthesia (topical) 31, 32, 36
anaphylaxis 69
audit 54-57

basic Life Support 68
blepharitis 65-67

cataract 43-45
choroid 4-6
choroidal neovascularisation (Classic) 22
choroidal neovascularisation (occult) 23
ciliary body 4-6, 10
clean room 61
clinical governance 54
collapse 42
consent 29, 30
cornea 3-5

endophthalmitis 48-50

fovea 6, 7
foveola 6, 7
fundus fluorescein angiography (FFA) 17

haemorrhage (subconjunctival) 42, 43
hyperfluorescence 21-24
hypofluorescence 25

intraocular pressure 42, 46, 47
iris 4, 5
ischemic optic neuropathy 46

leakage 19, 21, 23
lens 4, 5, 9, 10
long ciliary nerves 35

macula 6, 7
macular oedema (cystoid) 15, 23, 24
macular oedema (diabetic) 15, 16, 23, 24

masking   25, 27

occlusion (central retinal artery)   46
optical coherence tomography (OCT)   11

paracentesis   38
pattern (lacy)   22
pattern (petalloid)   24
pigment epithelial detachment (PED)   14, 23
pooling   20, 21, 23
povidone-iodine   31–34, 36, 39
pupil (dilation)   42–44

regurgitation test   65, 67
retina   3, 5–10
retinal detachment   46, 47

sclera   3–6

training   53–55

vitreous   9
vitreous detachment   9, 45

waste (anatomical)   59
wetlab   59
window defect   23, 26